TOXIC CONSTITUENTS OF ANIMAL FOODSTUFFS

FOOD SCIENCE AND TECHNOLOGY

A SERIES OF MONOGRAPHS

Maynard A. Amerine, Rose Marie Pangborn, and Edward B. Roessler, PRINCIPLES OF SENSORY EVALUATION OF FOOD. 1965.

C. R. Stumbo, THERMOBACTERIOLOGY IN FOOD PROCESSING, second edition. 1973.

Gerald Reed, ENZYMES IN FOOD PROCESSING. 1966.

S. M. Herschdoerfer, QUALITY CONTROL IN THE FOOD INDUSTRY. Volume I — 1967. Volume II — 1968. Volume III — 1972.

Hans Riemann, FOOD-BORNE INFECTIONS AND INTOXICATIONS. 1969.

Irvin E. Liener, TOXIC CONSTITUENTS OF PLANT FOODSTUFFS. 1969.

Martin Glicksman, GUM TECHNOLOGY IN THE FOOD INDUSTRY. 1970.

L. A. Goldblatt, AFLATOXIN. 1970.

Maynard A. Joslyn, METHODS IN FOOD ANALYSIS, second edition. 1970.

A. C. Hulme (ed.), THE BIOCHEMISTRY OF FRUITS AND THEIR PRODUCTS. Volume 1 — 1970. Volume 2 — 1971.

G. Ohloff and A. F. Thomas, GUSTATION AND OLFACTION. 1971.

George F. Stewart and Maynard A. Amerine, INTRODUCTION TO FOOD SCIENCE AND TECHNOLOGY. 1973.

IRVIN E. LIENER (ed.), TOXIC CONSTITUENTS OF ANIMAL FOODSTUFFS. 1974.

AARON A. ALTSCHUL (ed.), NEW PROTEIN FOODS: TECHNOLOGY 1A. 1974.

TOXIC CONSTITUENTS
OF ANIMAL FOODSTUFFS

Edited by

IRVIN E. LIENER

Department of Biochemistry
College of Biological Sciences
University of Minnesota
St. Paul, Minnesota

1974

ACADEMIC PRESS   New York and London
A Subsidiary of Harcourt Brace Jovanovich, Publishers

ACADEMIC PRESS, INC.
111 Fifth Avenue, New York, New York 10003

United Kingdom Edition published by
ACADEMIC PRESS, INC. (LONDON) LTD.
24/28 Oval Road, London NW1

Library of Congress Cataloging in Publication Data

Liener, Irvin E
  Toxic constituents of animal foodstuffs.

  (Food science and technology)
  Includes bibliographies.
   1. Animal food—Toxicology. 2. Food poisoning.
I. Title. [DNLM: 1. Food analysis. 2. Meat—
Poisoning. 3. Poultry products—Poisoning. QU50
L719t 1973 (P)]
RA1259.L53   615.9'54   73–2074
ISBN 0–12–449940–6

PRINTED IN THE UNITED STATES OF AMERICA

CONTENTS

3 Fish Eggs

Frederick A. Fuhrman

4 Shellfish, Fish, and Algae

Edward J. Schantz

5 Nitrosamines

N. P. Sen

LIST OF CONTRIBUTORS

Numbers in parenthesis indicate the pages on which the authors' contributions begin.

ROBERT E. FEENEY (39), Department of Food Science and Technology, University of California, Davis, California

FREDERICK A. FUHRMAN (73), Stanford University, Hopkins Marine Station, Pacific Grove, California

DAVID T. OSUGA (39), Department of Food Science and Technology, University of California, Davis, California

NORMAN SAPEIKA (1), Department of Pharmacology, University of Cape Town, Observatory, Cape, South Africa.

EDWARD J. SCHANTZ (111), Food Research Institute, University of Wisconsin, Madison, Wisconsin

N. P. SEN (131), Food Research Laboratories, Health Protection Branch, Department of National Health and Welfare, Ottawa, Canada.

PREFACE

We are living at a time when the public is becoming increasingly more concerned about the harmful effects of pollutants on the environment. Most of these pollutants are chemical in nature and are generated as by-products of a highly industrialized society. Some of these, of course, gain access, in one way or another, into our food chain where they may pose a threat to our health and well being. What is sometimes not fully realized, however, is that Nature herself has seen fit to introduce toxic substances into many of the foods which man consumes. It has been suggested that these toxic materials serve as a defense mechanism for the survival of certain species of plants and animals subject to predators (Whittaker and Feeny, 1971; Leopold and Ardrey, 1972). The potentially harmful effect of such substances in plant foodstuffs consumed by man and animals has been dealt with in a book, which may be considered a companion to this one, entitled "Toxic Constituents of Plant Foods" (Liener, 1969). Examples of naturally occurring toxicants in animal tissues used as food by man, on the other hand, are few in number, if for no other reason that it makes very little evolutionary sense to expect an animal organism to be genetically endowed with the seeds of its own destruction. However, if we include food additives, pesticides, chemical contaminants, etc.—i.e., substances of man-made origin—foodstuffs may then become a very significant vector for the dissemination of potentially toxic agents.

The subject of toxic factors in animal foodstuffs has generally been treated in a rather cursory fashion in more comprehensive treatises devoted to the general topic of naturally occurring toxicants (National Academy of Sciences, 1966; Gontzea and Sutzescu, 1968; Sapeika, 1969; Symposium, 1969). The object of this book is to treat the animal foodstuffs as a separate topic in which both aspects of the problem are considered, namely, those toxic substances which occur naturally as well as those which are deliberately or inadvertently introduced by man. The naturally occurring toxicants in animal tissue are, as mentioned before, limited in their distribution, and seem to be confined mainly to avian and fish eggs and to certain kinds of shellfish and amphibia. Examples of toxicity due to the introduction of man-made chemicals may be found in most meat and dairy products. In this connection, special consideration has been given to the timely problem of the carcinogenic nitrosamines in meat products to which nitrites have been added.

It is hoped that this book may bring to its readers an increased awareness of the fact that even products of animal origin may at times prove to be potentially hazardous to health because of certain toxic substances which, for a number of various and diverse reasons, may eventually find their way into such foods. Once the existence of these toxicants are recognized, there will be a vital need for their close surveillance in the food chain; this in turn will require new and improved techniques for their detection and their eventual elimination.

Irvin E. Liener

REFERENCES

Gontzea, I., and Sutzescu, P. (1968). "Natural Antinutritive Substances in Foodstuffs and Forages." Karger, Basel, 184 pp.

Leopold, A. C., and Ardrey, R. (1972). Toxic substances in plants and the food habits of early man. Science **176**, 512–514.

Liener, I. E. (1969). "Toxic Constituents of Plant Foodstuffs." Academic Press, New York, 500 pp.

National Academy of Sciences, National Research Council (1966). Toxicants Occurring Naturally in Foods." Publ. No. 1354, Washington, D.C.

Sapeika, N. (1969). "Food Pharmacology." Thomas, Springfield, Illinois, 183 pp.

Symposium on Natural Food Toxicants (1969). *J. Agr. Chem.* **17**, 413–538.

Whittaker, R. H., and Feeny, P. P. (1971). Allelochemics: chemical interactions between species. *Science* **171** 757–770.

1

□ □ □

MEAT AND DAIRY PRODUCTS

Norman Sapeika

I. Toxic Constituents of Meat

Meat is the flesh of warm-blooded animals used as food, the term usually excluding fish and poultry. The great majority of mankind has a natural appetite for meat; the flesh of more than 100 different species of animals is regularly eaten by man (Davidson and Passmore, 1969). However, vegetarians do not eat meat, fish, and poultry, although dairy produce and eggs are acceptable; "vegans" exclude also milk, butter, cheese, and eggs.

Most meat is eaten fresh, but great quantities are also salted, smoked, dried, canned, or preserved in other ways. Pemmican is well known as a preparation of dried meat from buffalo or beef which has been much used by hunters and explorers. It may induce nausea, but this mainly in those already suffering from starvation (Review, 1961a).

Meat extracts, for example, Bovril, contain amines which enter the bloodstream virtually unaltered in patients who are taking antidepressants of the monoamine oxidase inhibitor (MAOI) type such as tranylcypromine (Parnate), and phenelzine sulfate (Nardil). A dangerous rise in blood pressure can occur. Similar hypertensive episodes have occurred in patients receiving these drugs and who had eaten other tyramine-containing foods such as cheese, which is considered in Section IV.

A. ADDITIVES

Food additives include a great variety of substances that are intentionally added to enhance the appearance, taste, and structure, or the storage life of food. The shortage of food in the world, aggravated by the "population explosion," has further necessitated the use of substances that preserve food or diminish its wastage. This subject has been considered in many publications, for example, in Reports published by the Joint FAO/WHO Expert Committee on Food Additives, details of which can be obtained from Food Additives, World Health Organization, Avenue Appia, 1211 Geneva, Switzerland, or, Food Science and Technology Branch, Food and Agriculture Organization of the United Nations, 00100, Rome, Italy. Other publications that may be consulted are: Symposium on Additives and Residues in Human Foods (1961), National Academy of Sciences—National Research Council (1965, 1966), Extra Pharmacopoeia (1967), Philp (1968), Sapeika (1969),

Liener (1969), Roe (1970), and others referred to in relevant sections in this chapter.

Substances that may be added to food to act as preservatives are severely restricted by law in many countries. In the United Kingdom sodium nitrate is permitted in limited amounts in bacon, ham, and cooked meats (Sykes, 1965). Nitrates and nitrites have long been used in curing mixtures to make the visual appearance of meat attractive. This is due to their interaction with heme pigments. Nitrites also have an antibacterial action and retard decomposition of meat (Chichester and Tanner, 1968). The use of these substances in meat and meat products has occasionally caused poisoning (Steyn, 1960). An important finding is that nitrites (and nitrates) and certain other compounds, e.g., alkylureas present in meat, fish, and other foods, can lead to the formation of carcinogenic nitrosamides (Mirvish, 1971; Sander, 1971). Such compounds have been demonstrated to induce gastric carcinoma in animals at the site of local application. Nitrosamides formed in the stomach in man could be significant in the causation of gastric cancer. See Chapter 6 for more detailed coverage of this important subject.

Nicotinic acid and sodium nicotinate have also been used to preserve the red color in meat. According to Press and Yeager (1962) sodium nicotinate is added to millions of pounds of meat annually in the United States. It is used as an additive for both fresh and processed meats. They described endemic poisoning from this substance involving 44 students, and considered some other reported episodes of food poisoning due to nicotinic acid. The features included flushing and itching of the "blush area" of the face and neck, gastrointestinal symptoms, and sweating.

Antibacterial drugs added to meat to act as a preservative include antibiotics such as the tetracyclines, which are useful in preventing the bacterial spoilage of meat, poultry, and fish.

Sulfur dioxide also has long been used in meat and many other foods.

Polyphosphates are used extensively in the food industry, for example, in meat, soup thickeners, and cheese. Datta et al. (1962) suggest that the acceptable human daily intake for phosphate is about 420 mg/day for an adult man of 70 kg body weight.

A number of old and some of the newer additives and other chemicals in animal feeds which leave residues in food prepared from livestock and poultry were considered by Bird (1961).

Stilbestrol, which is a synthetic nonsteroid estrogen, is known to be carcinogenic. The possible hazards of its administration have recently been reported and discussed (Leading Article, 1971b). The possible effects of stilbestrol residue in meat are also under investigation. Apparently, since 1954, 75% of cattle in America have been fed stilbestrol to increase their weight, but in Sweden and other countries the feeding of this substance to cattle has been banned. In Britain it has been used on a small scale to fatten veal and some poultry, having been passed as safe under the Voluntary Veterinary Products Safety Protection Scheme; a different view may be taken by the Veterinary Products Committee of the Medicines Commission which has superseded the former body.

Selenium is present in appreciable amounts in meats, seafoods, and most grains (Schroeder et al., 1970). This trace element is essential for mammals, but, because of possible toxicity from residue in food animals, it should probably not be added routinely to animal feedstuffs. The ingestion of certain fodder and grain rich in selenium can produce poisoning in animals (Frost, 1960; Brown and de Wet, 1967); the condition is known as blind staggers or alkali disease. Although under some conditions selenium is carcinogenic in rats, no recorded case of human or animal cancer is known which could be attributed to environmental selenium.

The preservation of food by radiation treatment is now being widely used, for example, in the United States for military defense purposes and for civilian economy, in England for the treatment of meats and meat products, and in several European countries for their own particular needs (Sykes, 1965). Complete sterilization would be ideal but, since the dose required would generally be so high as to damage the appearance and nutritional properties of the food, a lesser degree of radiation, "radiopasteurization," is used for red and white meats and for certain other foods. There is no acquired radioactivity from such treatment. However, the fact that a small residuum of viable bacteria persists may permit a type of spoilage that is different from that which normally occurs because of the different nature and balance of the bacterial flora before and after treatment. Also, since radiopasteurization is less effective against enzymes than against bacteria, destructive enzyme action can proceed.

Off-flavors induced by radiation changes in meat proteins are most marked in beef, less in lamb and veal, and least in pork and chicken and some fish products.

B. Contaminants

1. Plant substances

Food contaminants, or harmful impurities, in meat and dairy products may have gained entry into the food directly or indirectly: (a) consumption by the animal of plants containing naturally occurring toxic substances; (b) from the direct application of pesticides to plants that are eaten by the animal; (c) from contamination of the soil by pesticides applied to plants, or from chemicals added to the soil itself, or from the presence in the soil of radionuclides; (d) from the incorporation of drugs in animal feeds designed to promote growth, for example, antibiotics; (e) from the preparation of food with additives that may contain harmful substances; (f) from drugs administered in the prevention and treatment of disease in animals, for example, pencillin in cow's milk; (g) from the use of pesticides including rodenticides in places where food is stored, for example, in cow stalls and barns; (h) from substances in food containers.

Meat that has been roasted or grilled on wooden skewers derived from the ornamental shrub *Nerium oleander* (Ceylon rose) has caused death from ingestion of the cardioactive (digitalis) glycosides (Watt and Breyer-Brandwyk, 1962).

In South Africa there is a disease known as *krimpsiekte* or "cotyledonosis." It has occurred in animals such as sheep and goats, and in dogs and human beings, for example, Bushmen, who had eaten the raw or undercooked meat or blood of poisoned animals (Sapeika, 1936; Watt and Breyer-Brandwyk, 1962).

It is of interest that the meat of the quail, a game bird related to the partridge and grouse, has on a number of occasions been poisonous. This has been attributed to the birds eating toxic plants such as hemlock, which does not affect them but which renders their meat toxic. During their wanderings in the desert the Hebrews ate manna and quail; an explanation for the availability of these foods is given by Keller (1957) and the acute fatal poisoning in many who ate this food is considered by van Veen (1966). The quail "fell in great profusion around the camp of the Israelites" and the numerous deaths associated with the consumption of these birds is mentioned in the Old Testament (Numbers 11). Symptoms developed quickly: "While the meat was yet between their teeth, before it was consumed. . . ." In recent years a number of people on the island of Lesbos have developed an acute myoglobinuric syndrome shortly after eating quail. This occurred in individuals sensitive to a substance present in the quail and which is regarded as the eliciting factor. Muscular fatigue is regarded as important since the disorder rarely occurs in persons at rest. This occurrence has been reported by Ouzounellis (1970), who suggests this explanation for the deaths of the Hebrews who were certainly in a state of fatigue from their efforts to collect as many quails as possible which they dried for use as food. However, myoglobinuria is also occasionally encountered in normal subjects, for example, in military trainees after severe exertion (Greenberg and Arneson, 1967), also in Haff disease (epidemics of which have occurred in eastern Europe possibly from an unidentified toxic substance present in contaminated fish), and in a variety of other disturbances involving muscle.

2. *Pesticides*

Pesticide residues in food of animal origin, especially in adipose tissues, form the main source of intake for man, therefore residue tolerances have been established by governments and the examination of residues in crops and foods is constantly being carried out. Food generally is the main source of exposure of the general population to organochlorine insecticides. Market basket surveys in the United States and the United Kingdom have shown that especially fat-containing foods such as meat, fat, milk, and butter, form the main dietary source of these compounds (Jager, 1970). The insecticide residue levels in food in the United States has not been increasing (Duggan and Wetherwax, 1967; Hoffman, 1968), and in the United Kingdom the residues are declining (McGill *et al.,* 1969).

Halogen hydrocarbon insecticides, for example, DDT, have been widely used for many years, but recently attempts have been made to restrict their use. This is because of fears regarding the significance to man of storage of these poisons in body fat. Also important are the possible effects of starvation on these body stores since it has been demonstrated in animals that acute DDT poisoning can occur from the sudden release of the toxic principles from the storage sites (Dale *et al.,* 1962; Gleason *et al.,* 1969).

The storage of halogenated hydrocarbon pesticides in the body fat in man, as well as in animals, is well established. The entry of these chemicals into the body is derived from many sources (Review, 1967b). Foods of animal origin such as milk, eggs, and seafood represent one source. There is no convincing evidence of any toxic, carcinogenic, or teratogenic effects of pesticide residues in man.

In the case of DDT concentration the damage is particularly serious in the higher carnivores. Although conspicuous mortality is not generally observed this is no guarantee of safety, as low concentrations may inhibit reproduction and thus cause the species to fade away (Woodwell, 1967). DDT has been banned for most purposes in recent years in a number of countries, although there is no firm evidence that it is proving harmful to man. The current view is that the use of DDT should be limited, but the controlled utilization of this and some other organochlorine pesticides is essential in the present state of knowledge (World Health Organization, 1970b).

Cooking does not have much effect in diminishing the DDT level in such tissues as pork or beef. Carter *et al.* (1948) fed beef cattle hay containing DDT and subsequently examined portions of meat before and after different methods of cooking, roasting, broiling, pressure cooking, braising, and frying. The DDT was not materially decomposed or lost as a result of these various heat treatments.

The use of mercury compounds as a pesticide in grain has caused poisoning in persons who had eaten the meat of animals that had consumed the contaminated grain.

3. Radionuclides

Research programs of the U.S. Atomic Energy Commission and agencies of other nations, particularly Britain and the U.S.S.R., have studied the movement of radioactive debris of nuclear explosives, including the pathways along which the radioactive pollutants are distributed in plant and animal tissues. Arnold and Martell (1959) and others have given an account of the circulation and distribution of radioisotopes in man's environment and indicate the paths of entry by which fallout of fission products reaches human beings.

The half-life of strontium-90, a contaminant that in animals is concentrated in bone and milk, is 28 years; in the case of cesium-137, which accumulates in muscle, liver, spleen, and other soft tissues, it is 30 years; for iodine-131 it is 8 days. Since strontium-90 is lodged chiefly in bone it is not concentrated by passing from animal to animal. Cesium-137, which becomes widely distributed in all cells, is passed along to meat-eating animals and may accumulate in a chain of carnivores. Iodine-131 enters man mainly through ingestion of cow's milk and becomes concentrated in the thyroid gland where, in the course of some years, it may cause the formation of thyroid nodules (Woodwell, 1967). The danger to the thyroid of the fetus is that the gland may be partially or completely ablated after the 10th to 12th week of pregnancy; prior to this time the fetal thyroid shows little tendency to take up iodine-131.

Irradiation of certain foods has been deliberately used for some years as a method of preservation of such food. There is a vast amount of data on numerous types of irradiated foods which has provided no evidence of radiation-induced toxicity or carcinogenic effects, but this is a matter that is still under careful investigation (Kraybill and Whitehair, 1967).

The content of certain radionuclides in meat and milk products in subarctic regions such as Finland and Lapland has been intensively studied, for example, by Miettinen (1967). Very little radio-iodine appears in meat, which can never be regarded as dangerous from this point of view. In meat the dominant fission product will always be cesium-137, and three food chains of cesium-137 (in Lapland) are recognized: one leading from lichen to reindeer meat, one leading from plants such as sedges and horsetails to cow's meat and milk, and one leading from the fresh waters through plankton to fish.

4. Polycyclic Hydrocarbons

Broiled meat (steaks), barbecued ribs, and smoked fish prepared over an open fire become contaminated with carcinogens from soot and from the charred surface of the food (Hueper, 1962; Howard and Fazio, 1969). Complex polynuclear hydrocarbons, including benzpyrenes and benzanthracenes derived from the incomplete combustion of fat, have been demonstrated on the surface of charcoal-broiled meat. It is recommended that meat should not be broiled over the flames of burning fat; the fire should quickly be extinguished with water. Meat may be cooked by the heat from the coals and not by the fire of a barbecue.

The possibility of carcinogenesis from this source has been considered, for example, by Hueper (1961), Kraybill (1963), and in a review (1965b). There is evidence that the consumption of smoked meats, sausages, and fish, over prolonged periods may be a causal factor in the development of cancer of the alimentary canal especially the stomach. Gastric carcinoma is common in the population of Iceland (Dungal, 1961) where it is the practice in rural areas to preserve mutton and fish by a heavy smoking process. These foods contain a significant amount of the carcinogen, 3,4-benzpyrene, as well as other compounds. Home-smoked food is apt to contain much higher amounts of polycyclic hydrocarbons, including 3,4-benzpyrene, than commercially smoked food (Thorsteinson, 1969). This is due to differences in intensity and duration of exposure of meat in the course of smoke curing processes. By filtering the smoke the contents of 3,4-benzpyrene and other polycyclic hydrocarbons in the smoked food can be significantly reduced without markedly impairing the curing capacity of the smoke.

The concentration of polycyclic aromatic hydrocarbons in various smoked foods was investigated by Bailey and Dungal (1958) and by Dungal (1961); for mutton they reported the following: acenaphthylene, 137.7; fluorene, 20.6; phenanthrene, 86.5; anthracene, 19.8; pyrene, 5.9; fluoranthene, 4.6; 1,2-benzpyrene, 0; 3,4-benzpyrene, 1.3; values expressed in μg/kg wet material, minimum values.

The presence of polynuclear hydrocarbons in smoked and roasted foodstuffs has also been reported by other investigators (Review, 1965b); for example, Lijinsky and Shubik (1965) isolated the following compounds (μg/kg of charcoal-broiled steak prepared in the laboratory): benzo(a)pyrene, 8; fluoranthene, 20; pyrene, 18; and chrysene, coronene, anthracene, and benzo(b)-chrysene in amounts varying from 0.5 to 4.5 Most of the polynuclear hydrocarbons were present in higher concentrations in steaks and barbecued ribs prepared in a restaurant. The amounts present in these broiled foods are small and do not necessarily constitute a danger to the consumers of such foods (Review, 1965b).

5. Antibiotics

Antibiotic contaminants may be present in food because of five possibilities (Garrod, 1965): (a) naturally present, as in the preparation of cheese; (b) added as preservatives of flesh foods, for example, tetracyclines in butchers' meat (permitted in the Argentine), in eviscerated poultry (permitted in Canada and United States); (c) supplement in animal feed; (d) prevention or treatment of intestinal infections in animals; (e) treatment of bovine mastitis. Antibiotics in milk and other food have disadvantages with regard to human health, as is well recognized in the case of penicillin hypersensitivity reactions.

6. Carcinogens

A number and variety of naturally occurring substances are carcinogenic in certain animals; these dietary carcinogens include the aflatoxins, the pyrrolizidine alkaloids, and the aliphatic azoxy glycosides, which are potently carcinogenic in rodents. Many investigators have given much attention to the chemical identification and pathogenic effects of these neoplastic agents that are liable to be present in foods in certain parts of the world. At the present time there is little definite evidence that aflatoxins in human diets are responsible for liver disease or tumors, but there is need for additional work on the effect of these mycotoxins in man. Attention is drawn in subsequent sections of this chapter to the mycotoxins and the possibility of carcinogens being formed in food as a result of the use of certain additives, e.g., nitrates, or certain methods of preparing food, e.g., broiling and curing meat.

II. Toxic Constituents of Liver

A. HYPERVITAMINOSIS A

Liver is a useful food that contains naturally a great variety of substances including certain vitamins and antianemic factors. However, there are circumstances where liver can be harmful and dangerous to life.

The livers of certain animals are very rich in vitamin A, and acute intoxication (hypervitaminosis A) has occurred in man, for example, in Arctic explorers, and in dogs, from the consumption of this material. The features that may arise from acute and chronic vitamin A poisoning are described by Dalderup (1968). Drowsiness, headache, vomiting, shedding of skin, and many other adverse effects can occur. The livers of polar bears, the Arctic fox, seals, whales, and sharks can be poisonous to man, presumably because of their high concentration of vitamin A. The amounts of vitamin A and other substances in liver and other foods are given in

TABLE I
Amounts of Vitamin A in Several Livers and Butter

	Vitamin A (IU per 100 gm fresh weight)
Liver	
Polar bear	1.8 million
Seal	1.3 million
Sheep or ox	4000–45,000
Butter	2400–4000

Documenta Geigy—Scientific Tables (1962) and by Hawk (1965). A few examples are given in Table I.

Recently Cleland and Southcott (1969) presented the histories of a number of persons who became ill following the eating of the liver of the hair seal or sea lion. The clinical features were regarded as compatible with a diagnosis of hypervitaminosis A. These authors refer to the literature dealing with illness following the ingestion of seal liver and compare the vitamin A content of this food with that of polar bear liver.

B. OTHER TOXIC CONSTITUENTS

Chicken liver, like certain other foods containing amines, for example, cheese (Section IV), may produce hypertension in patients receiving antidepressant drugs that are monoamine oxidase inhibitors.

The amount of estrogenic activity in liver is so small that a physiological effect in man is impossible.

Cesium-137 may be present in liver; this radionuclide, which has a half-life of 30 years, accumulates in soft tissues such as liver, muscle, and spleen.

III. Toxic Constituents of Milk

A. ALLERGY TO MILK AND MILK INTOLERANCE

Unlike naturally occurring food toxins, which are undesirable constituents that may produce effects in any individual who consumes them, allergens are usually normal food constituents that produce effects in certain individuals who have an altered reactivity or allergy to them; such substances are otherwise nontoxic. Almost any food can induce an allergic (antigen–antibody) reaction, and it is more common in the human infant than in the adult. Food allergy can give rise to many different clinical syndromes.

True allergy to cow's milk protein is probably very rare; Collins-Williams (1962) estimated that clinical sensitivity to it occurs in 0.3–7% of all children. Allergy to cows' milk protein is an often diagnosed, but rarely proven, abnormality, though well-authenticated cases undoubtedly exist. In severe cases even small amounts of cow's milk protein produce fulminating vomiting and diarrhea. The chemistry of milk proteins is complicated, and it is therefore difficult to determine which of the many milk proteins may be giving rise to symptoms (Frankland, 1970).

Antibodies to cow's milk and its fractions have repeatedly been demonstrated by various techniques to be present in the serum of infants, children, and adults (Mansmann, 1966); however, in infants' sera analyzed for cow's milk antibodies by hemagglutination, antibodies against human milk proteins have not been detected. Wright *et al.* (1962) estimated the levels of circulating antibodies to cow's milk proteins (bovine serum albumin and lactalbumin); a conspicuous finding was the lack of close correlation between the titers of maternal and cord blood.

In certain diseases of the alimentary tract abnormally high concentrations of circulating antibodies to cow's milk proteins may occur, for example, in patients with ulcerative colitis, coeliac disease, and idiopathic steatorrhea. These high antibody titers might indicate that in certain alimentary disorders abnormal absorption of such proteins occurs with enhanced antibody formation, or they might be an expression of previous hypersensitization to common dietary proteins which may serve as causal factors in these diseases (Wright *et al.*, 1962; Annotation, 1964). In patients with ulcerative colitis milk is usually well tolerated, but there are some patients who are sensitive to milk protein; whether this type of reaction indicates the cause of the condition or whether the inflammatory process allows the passage of a foreign protein into the bloodstream, inducing the formation of antibodies, is not certain.

The circulating antibodies have not been related clinically with sensitivity reactions to milk (Review, 1965c; Mansmann, 1966).

Many investigators have studied milk intolerance, which may be the cause of a variety of symptoms. The milk precipitin syndrome, with features of iron deficiency anemia, hepatosplenomegaly, poor growth, pulmonary hemosiderosis, gastrointestinal and atopic symptoms, appears to be associated with a milk antigen–antibody reaction (Heiner *et al.*, 1962; Mansmann, 1966). The suggestion has been made that sudden unexplained death in infants may on occasion be the result of a milk antigen–antibody reaction (Review, 1969).

Sensitivity to cow's milk has been considered in a report from the Council on Foods and Nutrition, A.M.A. (Heiner *et al.,* 1964). It was pointed out that the syndrome is difficult to recognize or to ascribe to any one constituent of the food, and it was indicated that there is evidence that the ingestion of cow's milk may cause the occult loss of significant amounts of blood into the gastrointestinal tracts of some children with hypochromic microcytic anemia.

There is no doubt of the existence of true milk intolerance in some individuals, particularly in infants and children (Review, 1969); symptoms may be severe, and a prompt response may occur to a milk-free diet.

Bronchial asthma in children may be based on immunological milk intolerance (allergen–reagin reaction); biochemical changes such as an increase in the extracellular fluid volume have been observed in addition to the clinical symptoms.

Since cow's milk used for infant feeding may be responsible for allergies to the milk and to other forms of intolerance, the milk from other animals, hydrolyzed casein, and soya preparations have been examined as possible substitutes. However it must be realized that synthetic milks and foods for infants are likely to be deficient in nutrients, even when attempts are made to restore these (Mann *et al.,* 1965). These foods also may be harmful in infants who have phenylketonuria and galactosemia.

B. ESTROGENS

Estrogens in foods of animal and plant origin are considered by Stob (1966). These substances may be present to some extent in cow's milk, especially in colostrum, which is not important as this material does not enter food products. There is evidence that the amount of estrogenic activity in cow's milk increases as pregnancy advances.

Bovine fat is normally nonestrogenic but, in animals as also in the human female, treatment with certain estrogens produces storage of estrogen in the body fat.

There is little danger that the consumption of milk or foods containing estrogenic activity will produce physiological changes in man.

C. TOXIC PLANT SUBSTANCES

A great variety of foreign substances have been demonstrated in cow's milk and in human milk; they may be derived from the ingestion of plants, drugs, or other chemicals (Sapeika, 1959; Sisodia and Stowe, 1964; Knowles, 1965; Extra Pharmacopoeia, 1967). Plant substances which gain entry into milk may produce minor or major unwanted effects. For example, the taste of onions or the smell of wild garlic or cod liver oil may be detectable in milk from cows that have eaten these substances.

1. Plant Goitrogens

Goitrogenic substances such as goitrin in cabbage, kale, turnips, rape seeds, and other plants, may pass into the milk of cows that eat these plants. This may cause interference with thyroid function in human beings who drink this milk (Clements, 1960; Wills, 1966). There is some evidence that thiocyanate may be the goitrogen in milk in certain parts of the world. A derivative of 2-thiooxazolidone has also been suspected as a goitrogen in cow's milk. Besides these two naturally occurring goitrogens there are many other possible goitrogens, some characterized as such, others not yet identified, although demonstrated to induce thyroid hyperplasia. The goitrogens that may be present in foods are reviewed by Wills (1966) and the significance of these substances in cow's milk is considered by van Etten (1969).

The goitrogenic activity of certain milks appears to be destroyed by heating or freezing the milk; ice cream, puddings, and other foods prepared from goitrogen-containing milk are much less active than the milk itself.

2. Other Toxic Plant Constituents

The plants known as white snakeroot and rayless goldenrod (jimmy weed) that grow in Texas, New Mexico, and Arizona, contain poisonous principles that cause the disorder in animals known as milk sickness, trembles, or alkali disease. Illness has also occurred in human beings who ingested the milk or meat of poisoned animals, as discovered originally by Dr. Anna Pierce Hobbs (Sniveley, 1966). The mother of Abraham Lincoln and several members of his family as well as many early settlers in North America died of this "milk sickness" (Locket, 1957). Severe gastrointestinal symptoms, prostration, liver damage with jaundice, renal damage with oliguria and anuria, hypoglycemia, ketosis, convulsions, and coma are produced; death occurs in 1 or 2 weeks. The leaves and stem of these toxic plants contain tremetol, an unsaturated alcohol $C_{16}H_{22}O_3$ which resembles turpentine in its consistency and odor. This poison inhibits the mobilization of glucose from liver glycogen. It is not inactivated by pasteurization of milk or milk products.

An infant that drank milk from a cow that had eaten the foliage of *Nerium oleander* L. allegedly died from this cause (Watt and Breyer-Brandwyk, 1962).

The juice from *Solanum incanum* has been used by Transkeian Bantu in South Africa to curdle milk. There is a high incidence of esophageal carcinoma in these people. Since dimethylnitrosamine (DMNA) has been identified in solanum fruit it is suggested that there may be a causative association between DMNA and other nitrosamines and this neoplasm (Du Plessis *et al.*, 1969). Nitrosamines are suspected as causal factors in human carcinogenesis because of the widespread occurrence of nitrosamine precursors in biological systems and the remarkable manner in which various nitrosamines can affect different organs in the same species of animal (Bonser, 1967). Certain compounds in meat can also lead to the formation of carcinogenic nitrosamides, as mentioned in an earlier section of this chapter and considered in detail in Chapter 5.

D. NITRATES, NITRITES, AND OTHER CONTAMINANTS IN INFANT FOODS

Feeding formulas for infants have caused poisoning in infants when toxic substances have inadvertently been added to the milk. The use of certain types of water containing nitrates, from wells or bore-holes, has caused poisoning and death from methemo-globinemia (Locket, 1957; Steyn, 1960); the low acidity in the stomach of infants may permit the growth of organisms that re-duce nitrate to nitrite which then converts the hemoglobin to methemoglobin. Knotek and Schmidt (1964), in Czechoslovakia, showed that alimentary methemoglobinemia in artificially fed in-fants is produced by nitrites originating from nitrates contained in water used in the dilution of dried-milk preparations. The reduc-tion of nitrates is induced by sporulating organisms (*B. subtilis*) con-tained as spores in the dried milk.

The accidental use of sodium nitrite present in antirust tablets, for the preparation of infant feeds, has caused similar poisoning.

Other substances that have been accidentally included in feeding formulas include boric acid. Babies have been given Dettol and water in mistake for milk, with fatal results.

The desirability of fluoridation of public water supplies is still a controversial subject. To avoid compulsory medication of this type, to which there is much opposition, alternative schemes have been devised; thus, in England the Borrow Dental Milk Foundation is investigating the use of precisely prepared fluoridized milk to prevent caries in children.

As far as human milk is concerned it is practically never necessary to remove a child from the breast when the mother is receiving drug therapy; this is borne out by the rarity of cases of untoward reactions reported in the literature. Most drugs given to the mother will appear in the milk but in low concentration and for a short period. This is due to the fact that many drugs given to the mother are bound to plasma protein, metabolized, or cleared from the body.

E. MILK–ALKALI SYNDROME

In patients with peptic ulcer who take large quantities of milk (which provides a high calcium diet), together with calcium car-bonate (absorbed as calcium chloride) and absorbable alkali such as sodium bicarbonate, there is risk of the development of the milk–alkali syndrome. Burnett and colleagues (1949) first described this syndrome of hypercalcemia and hypercalciuria, nausea, vomiting, abdominal pain, polyuria and thirst, uremia, and metastatic calcification in the arteries and kidneys. In advanced cases the cornea undergoes calcification, at first visible with the slit lamp and later recognizable with the naked eye (Locket, 1957).

F. ANTIBIOTICS

Antibiotics and other antimicrobial agents used in treating bovine disease, such as mastitis, gain entry into the cow's milk. More than 75 tons of antibiotics are used each year in the prevention or treatment of mastitis in the dairy cow. Penicillin is mostly used, but bacitracin, tetracyclines, and streptomycin are also employed. This practice is undesirable not only because of adverse reactions that may occur in individuals drinking such milk but also because of interference with the manufacture of cultured dairy products such as cheese and yoghurt (Freedman and Meara, 1959).

It is well established that penicillin is a common cause of drug allergy, and sensitive patients are warned to avoid receiving this antibiotic; even minute amounts have caused allergic reactions in such persons (Meyler and Herxheimer, 1968). Siegel (1959) has drawn attention to the many different ways in which persons may become exposed to this drug, including the ingestion of penicillin in contaminated milk. The Food and Drug Administration of the United States of America quickly recognized that such contaminated milk might be a health hazard to the consumer. Dairy farmers have been obligated to discard milk ordinarily distributed for human consumption for at least 3 days following the use of antibiotics.

Many drugs including antibiotics taken during lactation are excreted in the mother's milk (Sapeika, 1959; Knowles, 1965). Antibiotic residues in milk and cheese and the possible hazards were considered by an Expert Committee (World Health Organization, 1963, 1970a).

G. PESTICIDES

Cow's milk and human milk may contain pesticides (Sapeika, 1959; Review, 1960c; Leading Article, 1965; Egan et al., 1965) which may eventually find their way into body tissues. Egan *et al.* (1965) examined samples of human perirenal fat obtained at autopsy, also biopsy specimens and human breast milk, for various organochlorine pesticide residues derived from sources throughout England and Wales. The levels in the fat ranged from 0.2 to 8.5 ppm for total DDT equivalent (mean 3.3), from a trace to 1 ppm for total benzene hexachloride (BHC) (mean 0.42), and from a trace to 0.9 ppm for Dieldrin (mean 0.26). In human breast milk the corresponding figures were 0.075–0.170 for total DDT equivalent, 0.009–0.033 for total BHC, and 0.002–0.013 for Dieldrin.

Very low residues of organochlorine pesticides were found in milk, butter, beef fat, mutton fat, and corned beef produced or imported into Britain in 1963 and 1964, although some butter samples contained up to 0.1 ppm of DDT and 0.4 ppm of total DDT equivalent (Egan *et al.*, 1966; Lee, 1966).

H. RADIONUCLIDES

There is much literature dealing with the demonstration and estimation of radionuclides in cow's milk.

As in the case of meat, milk from animals that have eaten contaminated radioactive herbage presents a danger to man. There has been much investigation in recent years in this important special field of food and environmental pollution.

At different times cow's milk may contain radioactive substances, but a nursing mother who drinks such milk will not have significant amounts of radionuclides in her breast milk, and the intake of the baby is not a matter for concern (Note, 1961).

It was estimated in 1958 that in the United Kingdom milk, cream, and cheese contributed 65.7% of the strontium-90 ingested in the diet; in the United States in 1959, milk and milk products contributed 39% of the strontium-90 ingested. Useful as this information may be it is clear that milk alone is not a reliable index of strontium-90 content of the total diet.

The average contents of strontium-90 and cesium-137 in North American milk were published by Kulp *et al.* (1961), and, in the United Kingdom, the Agricultural Research Council Radiobiological Laboratory has examined the mean iodine-131 content of daily milk samples. There were found to be regional differences that resulted from climatic and geographic factors and from differences in the diet of cattle (Report, 1961).

Perkins and Nielsen (1965) measured the concentrations of sodium-22, cesium-134, and cesium-137 in several foods: meat, Alaskan caribou, moose, reindeer meat, and milk, and, in bioassay samples, from Alaskan Eskimos. They suggest that the same foods which carry cesium-137 to man are also the main sources of sodium-22. Hvinden and Lillegraven (1966) measured the radionuclides cesium-137 and strontium-90 in Norwegian milk from 1956 onward and found seasonal variations and variations from district to district; the variations seemed to be more dependent on feeding conditions than on deposition.

The nuclear weapons test by the USSR in 1962 resulted in the appearance of iodine-131 in Swedish milk as demonstrated by Åberg (1967). Most of the iodine-131 liberated by a nuclear explosion becomes inactive in the upper atmosphere, but the iodine-131 which falls on the pasture on which cattle feed passes readily into their milk. Thus far the level of contamination of milk does not appear to have caused any risk to the thyroid gland.

The concentration of strontium-90 in milk in the northern hemisphere increased temporarily as the result of nuclear weapons testing; plant foods may, however, contribute much more radioactive strontium to the diet of an adult than does milk.

Strontium-90 is an isotope with a half-life of approximately 20 years and, like certain other radionuclides, it proceeds through the food chain—soil to plants to meat and milk and its products—to the diet of man, whence it passes with calcium into the tissues and bone mineral (Review, 1961b,d,e, 1963).

Strontium-90 and cesium-137 in Canadian milk examined during the period 1960–1964 were consistently at levels higher than those in milk in the United States and Britain. Radioactive fallout of cesium-137 in the Canadian North resulted in this substance being retained (preferentially) in lichens and other plant materials; as these are the principal food items for reindeer and caribou at certain times of the year, the meat of these animals has become heavily contaminated with radionuclides. Eskimo in the Canadian North who consume such meat have been found, by techniques involving whole-body counts and urine examination, to have high cesium-137 levels (Bird, 1966; Woodwell, 1967).

Strontium resembles calcium in its chemical properties, and, like calcium, it is deposited in bone when it enters the body. However, the relative concentration when deposited in bone is different from their relative concentration in the diet. The deposition of strontium-90 in bone is related to the calcium content in the diet—the less calcium, the more strontium-90 is deposited. As milk is rich in calcium the body assimilates calcium and discriminates against the strontium. Should the diet be deficient in calcium, then relatively more strontium-90 is absorbed. In areas where people use little or no milk the strontium-90 in their bones is about as much as that in people in the United States, probably because of less calcium in their diet (Lampert, 1965).

The strontium-90 content of bone samples from South Africans of different race and age groups was investigated by van As and Fourie (1971). Whites and Bantu have different dietary habits and consequently different calcium intakes and sources of strontium-90 in their diets; the diet of Whites consists of 75% animal products and 25% cereals and of the Bantu 70% cereals and 30% animal products.

The average milk consumption of Whites in 1966 was 180 kg/year, and it formed 50% of the total strontium-90 intake. Although responsible for only 5% of the total calcium intake, maize may contribute up to 50% of the strontium-90 intake; a very important part of the daily Bantu diet is maize porridge. Significant differences were found especially in the age group 5–20 years. It appears that the strontium-90 contents in the bone of all the different population groups are inversely proportional to the total calcium in their diets and independent of the mode of strontium-90 intake.

Values for the radium-226 content (pCi/year) of milk, meat, and certain other foodstuffs collected in certain regions of America as given by Comar (1966) are shown in Table II.

The content of certain radionuclides in milk and meat products in regions such as Finland and Lapland is given by Miettinen (1967). Here too, as in the Canadian North, there is a food chain of cesium-137 from lichen to reindeer meat, also from grasses and plants such as sedges and horsetails to cow's meat and milk.

TABLE II
Radium-226 Content (pCi/year) of Some Foodstuffs in United States

	New York City	Chicago	San Francisco
Milk	50.8	46.4	46.4
Meat, eggs, poultry, fish	140.6	134.2	102.0

Godfrey and Vennart (1968) using a whole-body counter, measured the amounts of radiation from fallout cesium-137 in the bodies of a number of people in a heavily populated region, chiefly in the southeast corner of England. The principal sources of the cesium were milk, dairy products, and meat. The food consumed would not be markedly different from the average for the country except in the case of milk which tends to vary to a large extent in its place of origin for different consumers. The total radiation dose of cesium-137 was about 10 mrads for women and babies and about 50% more for men; the United Nations Scientific Committee reported in 1966 that 15 mrads was the average dose commitment from cesium-137 as the result of nuclear weapons testing prior to that date (cited by Godfrey and Vennart, 1968).

There is no evidence that the amounts of radioactivity present naturally in the diet and in the body is significant or deleterious. However, the natural background of radiation is important in view of addition of radioactivity to the biosphere and foodstuffs resulting from tests of nuclear weapons and the expanding uses of atomic energy.

I. MYCOTOXINS

Fungal toxins (mycotoxins) have been demonstrated in cow's milk. The presence of such substances, which in most cases have been demonstrated to be potent carcinogens in experimental animals, is obviously a matter of great concern to man where milk is used as food (Petering, 1966). Cows that have eaten aflatoxin-containing material eliminate some toxin in the milk, but not in easily detectable amounts in bulk milk supplies, presumably because of much dilution.

It was demonstrated by Allcroft and Carnaghan (1963) that extracts of the milk from cows that ate aflatoxin-containing seed proteins and other feeds can induce toxic effects in ducklings. De Iongh *et al.* (1964) also demonstrated the presence of a factor, toxic to the liver of ducklings, in the milk of cows that had been fed concentrate rations containing 15% of a highly toxic aflatoxin-containing groundnut meal. More recently Purchase and Vorster (1968) were able to detect the presence of aflatoxin M in milk samples purchased from retail commercial outlets in various towns. Aflatoxin M is a metabolite of aflatoxin when the lactating animal is fed an aflatoxin-containing diet. They point out that the most likely source of contamination of milk is the feeding of moldy groundnuts and groundnut hay to dairy cattle. Aflatoxin M is as significant to human health as is aflatoxin B in solid foods. This toxicological problem is considered in a report of the World Health Organization (1970a).

IV. Toxic Constituents of Cheese

Amines related to the aromatic amino acids occur in animal tissue and some are markedly pharmacoactive, for example, noradrenaline, adrenaline, and 5-hydroxytryptamine (serotonin). These compounds and others are also found in a variety of foods, such as certain cheeses, fruits, and vegetables.

It has been known for many years that cheese contains considerable quantities of amines. Their presence has more recently been demonstrated by modern chromatographic methods (Asatoor *et al.*, 1963).

The tyramine content of various foods was investigated by Horwitz *et al.* (1964); the amounts in various cheeses were as shown in Table III.

During ripening, the casein in cheese is broken down by rennet and bacterial action to form peptides and free amino acids. The concentration of tyrosine increases steadily as protein breakdown

TABLE III
Tyramine Content of Various Cheeses

Cheese	$\mu g/gm$
Camembert	86
Stilton	466
Brie	180
Emmentaler	225
New York State cheddar	1416
Gruyère	516
Processed American	50
Cream	Not detected
Cottage	Not detected

proceeds during maturation. Some of the bacteria produce amines, e.g., tyramine from tyrosine. The amount of tyramine in individual samples of the same type of cheese shows variations often as wide as those between different cheeses (Blackwell and Mabbitt, 1965). Foods subjected in their preparation to putrefactive microorganisms which decarboxylate amino acids will contain both monoamines and diamines. In cheese the conditions favor tyramine formation, but histamine is occasionally formed, and cadaverine and putrescine are often present in larger amounts (Blackwell *et al.*, 1965).

The amines in cheese are normally rapidly inactivated by monoamine oxidase, but in certain circumstances they may enter the body and produce adverse effects. In patients who are receiving antidepressant drugs of the monoamine oxidase inhibitor type (MAOI), for example, tranylcypromine, phenelzine, and nialamide, the inhibition of the enzyme in the intestine and liver may permit sufficient tyramine to escape oxidative deamination and enter the systemic circulation. Noradrenaline is then released from local stores, and also its action on adrenoreceptors becomes prolonged. As a result of this action a marked rise in blood pressure and other changes occur. Sudden severe throbbing headache is felt in the occipital region which may last many minutes, and even several hours. Death may occur in this hypertensive episode from intracranial hemorrhage. Such an attack has been produced by

28.5 gm (1 oz.) of cheddar cheese. Some clinical reports are referred to by Meyler and Herxheimer (1968).

The concentration of tyramine in Gruyère cheese has been found to vary from 11 to 1184 μg/gm (Price and Smith, 1971). The tyramine was unequally distributed in the cheese, most being close to the rind where it is probably derived from aerobic bacteria that grow near the surface of the cheese. These workers suggest this may explain why some patients receiving monoamine oxidase inhibitors (antidepressant drugs) report reactions to quite small amounts of cheese, while others find no effect at all after eating a large quantity of the same type of cheese. They also found that at the normal pH of saliva (6.5–7.0) about 5% of the tyramine content of the cheese may be absorbed from the mouth, thus bypassing intestinal and hepatic monoamine oxidase; if the tyramine content of a cheese is high, a sufficient amount could be absorbed to produce a systemic effect.

Other foods that have also produced hypertensive reactions in the presence of monoamine oxidase inhibitors include Bovril (a meat extract), chicken liver, pickled herring, Marmite, broad beans, and certain wines.

It is possible that attacks of migraine may be produced in certain persons by amines present in foods such as cheese and certain other foods (Hannington, 1967).

V. Toxic Constituents of Eggs

Eggs commonly cause allergic disorders such as urticaria and asthma in children and adults (Mansmann, 1966). In such individuals, eggs and foods such as biscuits and cakes which contain eggs must be excluded from the diet.

Egg albumin (egg white) has many constituents among which are the ovomucoids which inhibit trypsin (Ambrose, 1966) and a basic glycoprotein, avidin, which binds biotin, a member of the vitamin B group. When an egg is boiled these two potentially harmful constituents present in egg white are inactivated. A more detailed treatment of the toxic constituents of egg white may be found in Chapter 2.

Large amounts of egg albumin fed to animals produce diarrhea and loss of weight. In a man subsisting on a diet low in biotin the administration of raw egg white produces a dermatitis which is cured by biotin (Parsons, 1931; Williams, 1943).

Estrogenic activity has been demonstrated in the yolk of eggs but the amounts are insufficient to produce physiological effects.

The eggs derived from poultry that have been given antibiotics should not be sold for human consumption (World Health Organization, 1963).

Pesticides have been demonstrated to be present in the eggs of a number of species of birds because of the extensive spread of these chemicals in agriculture and horticulture (Dunachie and Fletcher, 1966). This has caused apprehension that some of these pesticides may have harmful effects on domesticated and wild animals.

Eggs may contain radioactive substances (Comar, 1966).

Egg yolk and animal fat contain most of the dietary cholesterol. These foods are considered important in the etiology of atherosclerosis which is discussed below.

VI. Atherosclerosis

The possibility of certain dietary constituents such as fats, sugar, and alcohol, being causal factors in the production and development of atherosclerosis has been much considered in recent years.

Analyses of the dietary fat content of different groups of individuals subject to different rates of coronary thrombosis have revealed some interactions, particularly with regard to international comparisons.

The total fat and cholesterol content (gm/100 gm edible uncooked food) of some meat and milk foods are given in Table IV.

Further details with regard to the above foods and many others are available in Documenta Geigy—Scientific Tables (1962) and Hawk (1965).

It would appear that there is a close association between atherosclerosis and a high plasma cholesterol determined by the quantity and quality of the dietary fat (Brock, 1961; Davidson and Passmore,

TABLE IV
Fat and Cholesterol Content of Some Meat and Milk Foods

	Fat (gm/100 gm)	Cholesterol (gm/100 gm)
Bacon	55–85	—
Ham	22–33	—
Milk	3.6	0.01
Butter	81	0.28
Cheese (cottage)	0.5	—
Cheese (other type)	25–36	0.13–0.19
Egg yolk (raw)	31.9	1.3

1969), but it remains to be proven that dietary factors and dietary measures influence the development of atherosclerosis in man.

A distinct correlation between arteriosclerotic disease and the ingestion of animal protein and saturated fats was demonstrated by Jolliffe and Archer (1959); fats considered to be saturated include beef, sheep, pig, eggs, cow's milk, cocoa bean, coconut, lard, and tallow. Diet is not the only factor but is an important consideration, and many workers have studied its influence on the incidence of coronary artery disease.

Saturated fats in the diet have been causally implicated by many other workers as an etiological factor in cardiovascular diseases. This has been proven by investigations in several animal species. Investigations indicate that polyunsaturated fats counteract, whereas saturated fats promote, atherogenesis. The plasma lipoprotein level can be changed by the type of dietary fat. The type of fat not only influences the total cholesterol content but also the free cholesterol, cholesterol esters, and phospholipids. Attention should be drawn to the possibility that adverse effects may result from the use of highly unsaturated fats to lower serum cholesterol; it has been suggested that the excessive consumption of such fats may be a causal factor of carcinoma of the stomach among the Japanese and Swedes (Harman, 1957).

There is a positive correlation between cholesterol and cholesterologenic dietary components and atherosclerotic disease of the coronary arteries (Review, 1960a, 1966). It is generally agreed that elevation of the serum cholesterol to a value greater than 250 mg/100 ml carries with it an increased risk of coronary arterial disease. Dietary regulation of serum cholesterol in man can diminish the risk of this disease (Review, 1967a), and several attempts have been made to measure the effect of lowering the serum cholesterol upon the risk of recurrence in patients who have had coronary thrombosis.

The lowering of cholesterol and the hyperlipidemia it often represents can in part be achieved by dietary management and by drugs. Levy *et al.* (1971) have presented in some detail the dietary management of the various types of hyperlipoproteinemia.

There is no proof as yet that lowering the serum cholesterol, reducing obesity, treating hypertension, or exercise improves the prognosis of survivors from an initial attack of coronary arterial disease, according to Jones (1970). Although the life-saving potential of serum cholesterol-lowering diets is not proven, the potential health benefits of these diets do not seem to be outweighed by any as yet unidentified hazards (Ederer *et al.*, 1971).

The Masai of East Africa have a staple diet of milk, meat, and blood. The average daily cholesterol intake is 500–2000 mg, which is comparable to the average in the United States. Despite their customary high-fat diet the aortas and coronary arteries of the Masai show little atherosclerosis. The serum levels of cholesterol, β-lipoprotein and pre-β-lipoprotein are low. In contrast to white people in the United States who have a limited maximal absorption capacity of 0.3 gm cholesterol the Masai can absorb more than 0.65 gm cholesterol. Compared with 25% suppression of synthesis found in the U.S. white people, the Masai can suppress 50% of their endogenous cholesterol synthesis. Investigators regard the Masai as having unique biological characteristics which are genetically determined and which protect them from the development of dietary induced hypercholesterolemia (Leading Article, 1971a).

It would appear that the dietary hypothesis of the etiology of coronary thrombosis has a base wider than cholesterol. It has been demonstrated, for instance, that a prediction of national mortalities from coronary thrombosis is given by their intakes of sugar (Yudkin, 1957, 1963). Cleave and Campbell (1966) and other workers have put forward the view that sugar and white flour consumed in large quantity over a prolonged period may be responsible for ischemic heart disease and a variety of other disorders.

Other hypotheses have also been put forward regarding atherogenesis, for example, that there is a deficiency of essential fatty acids, and that prostaglandins may play an important role in the effect of dietary fats (Thomasson, 1969).

Drinking water has also been incriminated. In England, for example, hard water compared with soft water in relation to the incidence of atherosclerosis has shown surprising differences; some association was found between softness of drinking water and increased death rates from cardiovascular diseases, although the foods consumed may be more important in determining the ultimate effects than the nature of the water (Review, 1967c,d, 1968). In Ontario, Canada, a detailed comparison of sudden deaths from ischemic heart disease was made by Anderson and le Riche (1971); they could establish no firm evidence of a real correlation between sudden death and either latitude or water hardness. According to Morton (1971a, b) the nitrate concentration is the water constituent most strongly associated with the hypertension risk pattern in Colorado.

Cardiovascular disease and certain other chronic diseases are more common in South India than in North India, and there are wide variations in the incidence rates of essential hypertension between the inhabitants of these areas; according to an investigation by Malhotra (1970), the differences appear to be due to hemodynamic changes probably induced by dietary factors (especially the long-chain vs. short-chain fatty acids in fats consumed) by virtue of their effect on the size and nature of chylomicrons, blood viscosity, and peripheral resistance.

Studies of Japanese who have emigrated to the United States indicate that the incidence of atherosclerotic heart disease is higher among the Nisei than among their relatives in Japan, while the incidence of cerebral hemorrhage and gastric carcinoma is lower. This change casts doubt on the role of genetics in the causation. It supports the concept that diet and/or some other environmental factor may be very important in this respect (Innami and Mickelsen, 1969).

VII. Foods Contraindicated in Certain Diseases

There are certain diseases in which naturally occurring food constituents may precipitate or aggravate the condition, or produce
other adverse effects. A few examples are given below of disorders
due to inborn errors of metabolism or to acquired diseases in which
certain food constituents must be avoided; if ingested they are
harmful or toxic to the patient.

Carbohydrate intolerance or malabsorption occurs in galactosemia, in essential fructose intolerance, and in certain other conditions such as gastroenteritis, coeliac disease, sprue, kwashiorkor,
chronic infection, or surgery in the neonate. Galactosemia may be
controlled in many affected infants if diagnosis is made early and a
lactose-free diet given; symptoms diminish when milk and milk
products are excluded from the diet (Hsia, 1967). There are
formulations of semisynthetic milk known as the Galactomins
(Drug and Therapeutics Bulletin, 1971) available for the treatment
of galactosemia and malabsorption of lactose or its constituents
glucose and galactose; however, skin eruptions and other evidences
of a deficiency state have been observed in galactosemic infants
receiving Galactomin (Mann *et al.*, 1965). The Galactomin powders
are a spray-dried blend of vegetable oils with liquid glucose or
fructose and partially demineralized cow's milk casein to which
vitamins and trace element supplements must be added. They are
unsuitable for infants intolerant of cow's milk protein.

Phenylketonuria (phenylpyruvic oligophrenia) is a disorder due
to an inborn error of amino acid metabolism; the basic defect is
the absence of the hepatic enzyme, phenylalanine hydroxylase,
which normally converts into tyrosine the dietary phenylalanine
that is not used up in the synthesis of protein. Mental deficiency
will occur unless the phenylalanine content of the diet is reduced
at an early age, for example, by the use of a phenylalanine-free
food such as casein hydrolysate (Review, 1961c,f). Proper dietary
management of this disease is not a simple matter; not only should
there be a balance between the intake of commercial low-
phenylalanine formula and natural foods, but the existence of diur-
nal variations in serum phenylalanine must be recognized (Review,
1970; Smith and Waisman, 1971).

Maple syrup urine disease, in which the urine has a characteristic odor, is an inborn error of the metabolism of branched-chain amino acids. The exclusion of valine, leucine, isoleucine, and methionine from the diet has produced some benefit (Review, 1965a).

In some patients with Crohn's disease (regional ileitis) milk seems to play a role in perpetuating disease activity and symptoms, and the effect of excluding milk from the diet for a few weeks should be observed. Also, in some patients who have diverticulitis coli or ulcerative colitis milk appears to precipitate diarrhea; this can be detected by the avoidance of milk for 1–3 weeks.

Milk and certain other foods may cause vomiting, borborygmi, diarrhea, and the dumping syndrome in some patients who have undergone a partial gastrectomy. This is due to the fact that the mucosal cells containing the enzyme that digests lactose are situated chiefly in the duodenum and upper jejunum, and these may be bypassed by gastrojejunostomy; inadequately absorbed lactose remaining in the intestine may then be fermented by bacteria.

In patients who have cirrhosis of the liver, and in a number of other disorders, the ingestion of nitrogen-containing compounds such as dietary protein or certain drugs produces a high concentration of ammonium ions in the blood. Neurological symptoms develop, progressing to stupor, coma, and death. This syndrome is known as hepatic coma or portacaval encephalopathy, and was previously called meat poisoning or ptomaine poisoning. The elimination of protein from the diet, emptying of the intestine by purgatives and enemas, and the use of antibiotics like colistin, kanamycin, and neomycin to prevent bacterial decomposition of food in the bowel, alleviates the condition (Review, 1960b).

In the treatment of interval gout patients have traditionally been advised to restrict the intake of foods rich in purine content, but strictly low-purine diets are no longer advocated.

In patients with hypoparathyroidism, where there is a decrease in serum calcium and an increase in plasma phosphate, foods such as milk, cheese, egg yolk, and certain others, are contraindicated as sources of calcium because of their rich content of phosphorus.

In allergic subjects the normal constituents of almost any food can induce an allergic reaction, giving rise to many different clinical syndromes. The reaction occurs in individuals who have an altered reactivity or allergy to such food constituents which are otherwise nontoxic.

There are certain foods that contain naturally occurring substances that may produce adverse effects when they are eaten at the same time as certain drugs are being administered. For example, as already pointed out, certain cheeses, chicken liver, and meat extracts contain amines such as tyramine that can produce hypertension in the presence of monoamine oxidase inhibitors. This is an example of drug interaction, which has become a serious problem in modern drug therapy.

Certain constituents of foods may be of importance in the causation of degenerative and other diseases. The best example of this is the possible relationship of dietary constituents to atherosclerosis and certain metabolic disorders. As already pointed out in a previous section, extensive evidence is available to indicate that elevated blood lipids are strongly associated with increased susceptibility to atherosclerosis and heart disease.

Dietary cholesterol and other fats have been found to favor the growth of certain malignant tumors in laboratory animals, and in man there are reports indicating a positive correlation between the consumption of fat and the occurrence of certain tumors (Review, 1967a). Before such correlations can be accepted there will need to be more evidence provided by fully controlled clinical and experimental studies.

References

Aberg, B. (1967). *In* "Minor Constituents in Foods" (J.C. Somogy; and P. Roine, eds.), pp. 32–42. Karger, Basel.

Allcroft, R., and Carnaghan, R.A. (1963). An examination for toxin in human food products from animals fed toxic peanut meal. *Vet. Res.* **75,** 259–263.

Ambrose, A.A. (1966) Naturally occurring antienzymes (inhibitors). *Nat. Acad. Sci.– Nat. Res. Counc., Publ.* **1354,** 105–111.

Anderson, T.W., and le Riche, W.H. (1971). Sudden death from ischemic heart disease in Ontario and its correlation with water hardness and other factors. *Can. Med. Ass. J.* **105,** 155–160.

Annotation. (1964). Antibodies and alimentary disease. *Brit. Med. J.* **2,** 328.

Arnold, J.R., and Martell, E.A. (1959). The circulation of radioactive isotopes. *Sci. Amer.* **201,** 85–93.

Asatoor, A.M., Levi, A.J., and Milne, M.D. (1963). Tranylcypromine and cheese. *Lancet* **2,** 733–734.

Bailey, E.J., and Dungal, N. (1958). Polycyclic hydrocarbons in Icelandic smoked foods. *Brit. J. Cancer* **12,** 348–350.

Bird, H.R. (1961). Additives and residues in foods of animal origin. *Amer. J. Clin. Nutr.* **9,** 260–268.

Bird, P.M. (1966). Radionuclides in foods. *Can. Med. Ass. J.* **94,** 590–597.

Blackwell, B., and Mabbitt, L.A. (1965). Tyramine in cheese related to hypertensive crises after monoamine-oxidase inhibition. *Lancet* **1,** 938–940.

Blackwell, B., Marley, E., and Mabbitt, L.A. (1965). Effects of yeast extract after monoamine oxidase inhibition. *Lancet* **1,** 940–943.

Bonser, G.M. (1967). Factors concerned in the location of human and experimental tumours. *Brit. Med. J.* **2,** 655–660.

Brock, J.F. (1961). "Recent Advances in Human Nutrition." Churchill, London.

Brown, J.M.M., and de Wet, P.J. (1967). A survey of the occurrence of potentially harmful amounts of selenium in the vegetation of the Karoo. *Onderstepoort J. Vet. Res.* **34,** 161–217.

Burnett, C.H., Commons, R.R., Albright, F., and Howard, J.E. (1949). Hypercalcaemia without hypercalcuria or hypophosphatemia, calcinosis and renal insufficiency. *N. Engl. J. Med.* **240,** 787–794.

Carter, R.H., Hubanks, P.E., Mann, H.D., Alexander, L.M., and Schopmeyer, G.E. (1948). Effect of cooking on the DDT content of beef. *Science* **107,** 347.

Chichester, D.F., and Tanner, F.W. (1968). Nitrites and nitrates. In "Handbook of Food Additives" (T.W. Furia, ed.). Chem. Rubber Publ. Co., Cleveland, Ohio.

Cleave, T.L., and Campbell, G.D. (1966). "Diabetes, Coronary Thrombosis, and Saccharine Disease." Wright, Bristol.

Cleland, J.B., and Southcott, R.V. (1969). Illnesses following the eating of seal liver in Australian waters. *Med. J. Aust.* **1,** 760–763.

Clements, F.W. (1960). Naturally occurring goitrogens. *Brit. Med. Bull.* **16,** 133–137.

Collins-Williams, C. (1962). Cow's milk allergy in infants and children. *Int. Arch. Allergy Appl. Immunol.* **20,** 38–59.

Comar, C.L. (1966). Natural radioactivity in the biosphere and foodstuffs, *Nat. Acad. Sci.–Nat. Res. Counc., Publ.* **1354,** 117–125.

Dalderup, C.B.M. (1968). In "Side Effects of Drugs" (L. Meyler and A. Herxheimer, eds.), Vol. VI, pp. 373–375. Excerpta Med. Found., Amsterdam.

Dale, W.E., Gaines, T.B., and Hayes, W.J. (1962). Storage and excretion of DDT in starved rats. *Toxicol. App. Pharmacol.* **4,** 89–106.

Datta, P.K., Frazer, A.C., Sharratt, M., and Sammons, H.G. (1962). Biological effects of food additives. II. Sodium pyrophosphate. *J. Sci. Food. Agr.* **13,** 556–566.

Davidson, S., and Passmore, R. (1969). "Human Nutrition and Dietetics." Livingstone, Edinburgh.

de Iongh, H., Vles, R.O., and van Pelt, J. G. (1964). Milk of mammals fed an aflatoxin-containing diet. *Nature (London),* **202,** 466–467.

Documenta Geigy—Scientific Tables, (1962). 6th ed., J.R. Geigy, S.A., Basel.

Drug and Therapeutics Bulletin (1971). The galactomins—semi-synthetic food powders. *Drug Ther. Bull.* **9,** 53–55.

Duggan, R.E., and Wetherwax, J.R. (1967). Dietary intake of pesticide residues. *Science* **157,** 1007–1010.

Dunachie, J.F., and Fletcher, W.W. (1966). Effect of some insecticides on the hatching rate of hen's eggs. *Nature (London)* **212,** 1062–1063.

Dungal, N. (1961). The special problem of stomach cancer in Iceland. *J. Amer. Med. Ass.* **178,** 789–798.

Du Plessis, L.S., Nunn, J.R., and Roach, W.A. (1969). Carcinogen in a Transkeian Bantu food additive. *Nature (London)* **222,** 1198–1199.

Ederer, F., Leren, P., Turpeinen, O., and Frantz, I.D.(1971). Cancer among men on cholesterol-lowering diets. *Lancet* **2,** 203–206.

Egan, H., Goulding, R., Roburn, J., and Tatton, J.O'G. (1965). Organochlorine pesticide residues in human fat and human milk. *Brit. Med. J.* **2,** 66–69.

Egan, H., Holmes, D.C., Roburn, J., and Tatton, J.O'G. (1966). Pesticide residues in foodstuffs in Great Britain. II. Persistent organochloride pesticide residues in selected food. *J. Sci. Food Agr.* **17,** 563–569.

Extra Pharmacopoeia (Martindale). (1967). Pharmaceutical Press, London.

Frankland, A.W. (1970). Food allergies. *Roy. Soc. Health, J.* **90,** 243–247.

Freedman, M.L., and Meara, P.J. (1959). Antibiotic contamination of milk supplies as a veterinary and public health problem. *S.A. Practitioner* **5,** 3–16.

Frost, D.V. (1960). Arsenic and selenium in relation to the Food Additive Law of 1958. *Nutr. Rev.* **18,** 129–132.

Garrod, L.P. (1965). Antibiotics in food. *Practitioner* **195,** 36–40.

Gleason, M.N., Gosselin, R.E., Hodge, H.C., and Smith, R.P. (1969). "Clinical Toxicology of Commercial Products." Williams & Wilkins, Baltimore, Maryland.

Godfrey, B.E., and Vennart, J. (1968). Measurements of caesium-137 in human beings in 1958–67. *Nature (London)* **218,** 741–746.

Greenberg, J., and Arneson, L. (1967). Exertional rhabdomyolysis with myoglobinuria in a large group of military trainees. *Neurology* **17,** 216–222.

Hannington, E. (1967). Preliminary report on tyramine headache. *Brit. Med. J.* **2,** 550–551.

Harman, D. (1957). Atherosclerosis: Possible ill-effects of the use of highly unsaturated fats to lower serum-cholesterol levels. *Lancet* **2,** 1116–1117.

Hawk, P.B. (1965). 'Physiological Chemistry, '4th ed. McGraw-Hill, New York.

Heiner, D.C., Sears, J.W., and Kniker, W.T. (1962). Multiple precipitins to cow's milk in chronic respiratory disease. *Amer. J. Dis. Child.* **103,** 634–654.

Heiner, D.C., Wilson, J.F., and Lahey, M.E. (1964). Sensitivity to cow's milk. *J. Amer. Med. Ass.* **189,** 563–567.

Hoffman, W.S. (1968). Clinical evaluation of the effects of pesticides on man. *Ind. Med. Surg.* **37,** 289–292.

Horwitz, D., Lovenberg, W., Engelman, K., and Sjoerdsma, A. (1964). Monoamine oxidase inhibitors, tyramine, and cheese. *J. Amer. Med. Ass.* **188,** 1108–1110.

Howard, J.W., and Fazio, T. (1969). A review of polycyclic aromatic hydrocarbons in foods. *J. Agr. Food Chem.* **17,** 527–538.

Hsia, Y. (1967). Clinical variants of galactosemia. *Metab. Clin. Exp.* **16**, 419–437.

Hueper, W.C. (1961). Carcinogens in the human environment. *Arch. Pathol.* **71**, 355–380.

Hueper, W.C. (1962). Environmental and occupational cancer hazards. *Clin. Pharmacol. Ther.* **3**, 776–813.

Hvinden, T., and Lillegraven, A. (1966). Caesium-137 and strontium-90 in Norwegian milk, 1960–1964. *Nature (London)* **210**, 580–583.

Innami, S., and Mickelsen, O. (1969). Nutritional status—Japan. *Nutr. Rev.* **27**, 275–278.

Jager, K.W. (1970). "Aldrin, Dieldrin, Endrin, and Telodrin." Elsevier, Amsterdam.

Jolliffe, N., and Archer, M. (1959). Statistical associations between international coronary heart disease death rates and certain environmental factors. *J. Chron. Dis.* **9**, 636–652.

Jones, A.M. (1970). The nature of the coronary problem. *Brit. Heart J.* **32**, 583–591.

Keller, W. (1957). "The Bible as History." Hodder & Stoughton, London.

Knotek, Z., and Schmidt, P. (1964). Pathogenesis, incidence, and possibilities of preventing alimentary nitrate methemoglobinaemia in infants. *Pediatrics* **34**, 78–83.

Knowles, J.A. (1965). Excretion of drugs in milk—a review. *J. Pediat.* **66**, 1068–1082.

Kraybill, H.F. (1963). Carcinogenesis associated with foods, food additives, food degradation products, and related dietary factors. *Clin., Pharmacol. Ther.* **4**, 73–87.

Kraybill, H.F., and Whitehair, L.A. (1967). Toxicological safety of irradiated foods. *Annu. Rev. Pharmacol.* **7**, 357–380.

Kulp, J.L., Schulert, A.R., Hodges, E.J., Anderson, E.C., and Langham, W.H. (1961). Strontium-90 and caesium-137 in North American milk. *Science* **133**, 1768–1770.

Lampert, L.M. (1965). "Modern Dairy Products." Chem. Publ. Co., New York.

Leading Article, (1965). Pesticides in the body. *Brit. Med. J.* **2**, 62.

Leading Article, (1971a). The Masai's cholesterol. *Brit. Med. J.* **3**, 262–263.

Leading Article, (1971b). Stilbestrol and cancer. *Brit. Med. J.* **3**, 593–594.

Lee, D.F. (1966). Pesticide residues in foodstuffs in Great Britain. I. Introduction. *J. Sci. Food Agr.* **17**, 561–562.

Levy, R.I., Bonnell, M., and Ernst, N.D. (1971). Dietary management of hyperlipoproteinaemia. *J. Amer. Diet. Ass.* **58**, 406–416.

Liener, I.E., ed. (1969). "Toxic Constituents of Plant Foodstuffs." Academic Press, New York.

Lijinski, W., and Shubik, P. (1965). Polynuclear hydrocarbon carcinogens in cooked meat and smoked food. *Ind. Med. Surg.* **34**, 152.

Locket, S. (1957). "Clinical Toxicology." Kimpton, London.

McGill, A.E.J., Robinson, J., and Stein, M. (1969). Residues of dieldrin (HEOD) in complete prepared meals in Great Britain during 1967. *Nature (London)* **221**, 761–762.

Malhotra, S.L. (1970). Dietary factors causing hypertension in India. *Amer. J. Clin. Nutr.* **23**, 1353–1363.

Mann, T.P., Wilson, K.M., and Clayton, B.E. (1965). A deficiency state arising in infants on synthetic foods. *Arch. Dis. Childhood* **40**, 364–375.

Mansmann, H.C. (1966). Foods as antigens and allergens. *Nat. Acad. Sci.–Nat. Res. Counc. Publ.* **1354**, 72–93.

Meyler, L., and Herxheimer, A. (1968). "Side Effects of Drugs." Excerpta Med. Found., Amsterdam.

Miettinen, D.D. (1967). *In* "Minor Constituents in Foods" (J.C. Somogyi and P. Roine, eds.), pp. 43–58. Karger, Basel.

Mirvish, S.S. (1971). Kinetics of nitrosamide formation from alkylureas, N-alkylurethans, and alkylguanidines: Possible implications for the etiology of human gastric cancer. *J. Nat. Cancer Inst.* **46**, 1183–1193.

Morton, W.E. (1971a). Hypertension and drinking water. *J. Chron. Dis.* **23**, 537–545.

Morton, W.E. (1971b). Hypertension and drinking water constituents in Colorado. *Amer. J. Pub. Health* **61**, 1371–1378.

National Academy of Sciences—National Research Council. (1965). "Chemicals Used in Food Processing," Pub. No. 1274. Nat. Acad. Sci.—Nat. Res. Counc., Washington, D.C.

National Academy of Sciences—National Research Council. (1966). "Food Protection Committee: Toxicants Occurring Naturally in Foods," Pub. No. 1354. Nat. Acad. Sci.—Nat. Res. Counc., Washington, D.C.

Note. (1961). Radioactive substances in breast milk. *Brit. Med. J.* **2**, 1375.

Ouzounellis, T. (1970). Some notes on quail poisoning. *J. Amer. Med. Ass.* **211**, 1186–1187.

Parsons, H.T. (1931). The physiological effect of diets rich in egg white. *J. Biol. Chem.* **90**, 351–367.

Perkins, R.W., and Nielsen, J.M. (1965). Sodium-22 and caesium-134 in foods, man and air. *Nature (London)* **205**, 866–867.

Petering, H.G. (1966). Foods and feeds as sources of carcinogenic factors. *Nutr. Rev.* **24**, 321–324.

Philp, J. McL. (1968). In "Modern Trends in Toxicology" (E. Boyland and R. Goulding, eds.), pp. 243–266. Butterworth, London.

Press, E., and Yeager, L. (1962). Food "poisoning" due to sodium nicotinate. *Amer. J. Publ. Health* **52**, 1720–1728.

Price, K., and Smith, S.E. (1971). Cheese reaction and tyramine. *Lancet* **1**, 130–131.

Purchase, I.F.H., and Vorster, L.J. (1968). Aflatoxin in commercial milk samples. *S. Afr. Med. J.* **42**, 219.

Report. (1961). Iodine-131 in milk. *Lancet* **2**, 1195–1196.

Review. (1960a). Coronary heart disease and dietary habits. *Nutr. Rev.* **18**, 9–11.

Review. (1960b). Hepatic coma. *Nutr. Rev.* **18**, 229–230.

Review. (1960c). Accumulation of insecticides in tissues and excretion in milk. *Nutr. Rev.* **18**, 235–237.

Review. (1961a). Pemmican. *Nutr. Rev.* **19**, 73–75.

Review. (1961b). Strontium-90 in the British diet. *Nutr. Rev.* **19**, 164–166.

Review. (1961c). Results of treatment in phenylketonuria. *Nutr. Rev.* **19**, 234–236.

Review. (1961d). Dietary components and accumulation of radionuclides in the body. *Nutr. Rev.* **19**, 245–247.

Review. (1961e). Radionuclides, calcium, and potassium in milk. *Nutr. Rev.* **19**, 253–254.

Review. (1961f). Phenylketonuria. *Nutr. Rev.* **19**, 264–266.

Review. (1963). Radionuclides in American diets. *Nutr. Rev.* **21**, 105–106.

Review. (1965a). Dietary treatment of maple syrup urine disease. *Nutr. Rev.* **23**, 260–262.

Review. (1965b). Hydrocarbon residues in cooked and smoked meats. *Nutr. Rev.* **23**, 268–270.

Review. (1965c). Antibody to milk proteins. *Nutr. Rev.* **23**, 299–301.

Review. (1966). Diet and coronary heart disease. *Nutr. Rev.* **24**, 228–230.

Review. (1967a). Dietary fat and neoplasms in man. *Nutr. Rev.* **25**, 8–9.

Review. (1967b). Dietary intake and fat storage of pesticides. *Nutr. Rev.* **25**, 68–71.

Review. (1967c). Diet and heart disease. *Nutr. Rev.* **25**, 130–132.

Review. (1967d). Atherosclerosis and the hardness of drinking water. *Nutr. Rev.* **25**, 164–166.

Review. (1968). Cardiovascular mortality and soft drinking water. *Nutr. Rev.* **26**, 295–297.

Review. (1969). Gastrointestinal milk allergy in infants. *Nutr. Rev.* **27**, 7–9.

Review. (1970). Growth and nutrition in treated phenylketonic patients. *Nutr. Rev.* **28**, 151–153.

Roe, F.J.C. (1970). "Metabolic Aspects of Food Safety." Blackwell, Oxford.

Sander, J. (1971). Compounds linked to cancer. *J. Amer. Med. Ass.* **216**, 1106–1108.

Sapeika, N. (1936). The pharmacological actions of plants of the genera Cotyledon and Crassula, N.O. Crassulaceae. *Arch. Int. Pharmocodyn. Ther.* **54**, 307–328.

Sapeika, N. (1959). The excretion of drugs, pesticides, and radionuclides in milk. *S. Afr. Med. J.* **33**, 818–820.

Sapeika, N. (1969). "Food Pharmacology." Thomas, Springfield, Illinois.

Schroeder, H.A., Frost, D.V., and Balassa, J.J. (1970). Essential trace metals in man: Selenium. *J. Chron. Dis.* **23**, 227–243.

Siegel, B.B. (1959). Hidden contacts with penicillin. *Bull. WHO* **21**, 703–713.

Sisodia, C.S., and Stowe, C.M. (1964). The mechanism of drug secretion into bovine milk. *Ann. N.Y. Acad. Sci.* **111**, 650–661.

Smith, B.A., and Waisman, H.A. (1971). Adequate phenylalanine diet for optimum growth and development in the treatment of phenylketonuria. *Amer. J. Clin. Nutr.* **24**, 423–431.

Sniveley, W.D. (1966). Discoverer of the cause of Milk Sickness. *J. Amer. Med. Ass.* **196**, 1055–1060.

Steyn, D.G. (1960). The problem of methaemoglobinaemia in man with special reference to poisoning with nitrates and nitrites in infants and children. *Univ. Pretoria Publ., Ser. 2.* **11**.

Stob, M. (1966). Estrogens in foods. *Nat. Acad. Sci.–Nat. Res. Counc., Publ.* **1354**, 18–23.

Sykes, G. (1965). "Disinfection and Sterilization." Spon, London.

Symposium on Additives and Residues in Human Foods. (1961). *Amer. J. Clin. Nutr.* **9**, 259–303.

Thomasson, H.J. (1969). Prostaglandins and cardiovascular disease. *Nutr. Rev.* **27**, 67–69.

Thorsteinson, T. (1969). Polycyclic hydrocarbons in commercially and home-smoked food in Iceland. *Cancer* **23**, 455–457.

van As, D., and Fourie, H.O. (1971). Strontium-90 in the bone of different South African population groups. *S. Afr. Med. J.* **45,** 694–696.

van Etten, C.H. (1969). Goitrogen *In* "Toxic Constituents of Plant Foodstuffs" (I.E. Liener, ed.), p. 103–142. Academic Press, New York.

van Veen, A.G. (1966). Toxic properties of some unusual foods. *Nat. Acad. Sci.– Nat. Res. Counc., Publ.* **1354,** 174–182.

Watt, J.M., and Breyer-Brandwyk, M.G. (1962). "The Medicinal and Poisonous Plants of Southern and Eastern Africa," 2nd ed. Livingstone, Edinburgh.

Williams, R.H. (1943). Clinical biotin deficiency. *N. Eng. J. Med.* **228,** 247–252.

Wills, J.H. (1966). Goitrogens in foods. *Nat. Acad. Sci.–Nat. Res. Counc., Publ.* **1354,** 3–17.

Woodwell, G.M. (1967). Toxic substances and ecological cycles. *Sci. Amer.* **216,** 24–31.

World Health Organization. (1963). The public health aspects of the use of antibiotics in food and feedstuffs. *World Health Organ., Tech. Rep. Ser.* **260**

World Health Organization. (1970a). Joint FAO-WHO expert committee on milk hygiene. *World Health Organ., Tech. Rep. Ser.* **453.**

World Health Organization. (1970b). Pesticide residues in food. *World Health Organ., Tech. Rep. Ser.* **458.**

Wright, R., Taylor, K.B., Truelove, S.C., and Aschaffenburg, R. (1962). Circulating antibodies to cow's milk proteins and gluten in the newborn. *Brit. Med. J.* **2,** 513–515.

Yudkin, J. (1957). Diet and coronary thrombosis—hypothesis and fact. *Lancet* **2,** 155–162.

Yudkin, J. (1963). Nutrition and palatability, with special reference to obesity, myocardial infarction, and other diseases of civilization. *Lancet* **1,** 1335–1340.

2

□ □ □

AVIAN EGG WHITES

David T. Osuga and Robert E. Feeney

I. Introduction

Avian egg-white constituents have been intensely investigated for many years by scientists with diverse interests. Probably the main reasons for this variety of interests have been the existence in avian egg whites of relatively high concentrations of proteins with differing biochemical properties, and the early observations that one of the proteins, avidin, complexes a B vitamin, and thereby may cause a nutritional deficiency in laboratory animals. The other egg-white proteins with complexing capacities or antimicrobial activities have also been suspected of possessing growth-inhibiting or toxic activities for animals.

Fortunately, there have been only a few reports of adverse effects from consumption of egg white by man, other than effects attributed to microbial or chemical contamination, or to allergic phenomena. In the case of avidin, egg white is seldom consumed in any quantity without the consumption of egg yolk and other foods containing adequate amounts of biotin; also the egg white is frequently heated sufficiently to inactivate the avidin. But another chicken egg-white protein, ovomucoid, was incorrectly incriminated as toxic to man, based on experiments with bovine materials. Only many years after discovery of the biochemical function of ovomucoid as an inhibitor of bovine trypsin was it proven (and accepted) that chicken ovomucoid does not inhibit human trypsin.

However, despite the paucity of evidence that chicken egg-white proteins are harmful to man as food constituents, the presence in egg white of over half a dozen proteins with particular properties capable of disrupting biochemical systems is perhaps ample reason for periodically summarizing what is known about these proteins. Such information might prevent the use of egg white in some hypothetical mixture or formula where these biochemically active proteins might be undesirable, but even this seems remote. Perhaps most important is to provide information so as to reduce the number of unsupported accusations (a popular pastime today!) of toxic effects of a wholesome food.

Egg white and egg-white constituents considered in this review will refer to those from the chicken *(Gallus gallus)* unless otherwise stated. The proteins which have been associated with adverse effects on man, other animals, or microorganisms are: (1) avidin, the protein responsible for "egg-white injury," and which binds 4 moles of biotin per mole of avidin; (2) ovomucoid, a mucoprotein which specifically inhibits an equal molar amount of bovine trypsin; (3)

ovoinhibitor, an inhibitor of several proteolytic enzymes; (4) ovo-transferrin, a metal-binding protein; (5) ovoflavoprotein (ovoapo-protein), a riboflavin-binding protein; (6) lysozyme, a carbohydrase capable of lysing certain microbial cells.

II. General Composition of Egg White

A. CHICKEN

Egg white is primarily a solution of proteins. The major charac-terized constituents, the amounts present, and some of their physical properties are listed in Table I. The remainder of the constituents include small amounts of various known proteins, un-identified proteins (mainly globulins), and nonprotein constituents (primarily glucose and salts).

Ovalbumin is the most abundant egg-white protein. The charac-teristic properties are that it is easily denatured, and contains most of the sulfhydryl groups present in egg white. A total of four SH groups per mole of ovalbumin were demonstrated to be present by MacDonnell et al. (1951). The total amount was detectable only after denaturation of ovalbumin and 1 to 3 of these groups will react with different chemical reagents (MacDonnell et al., 1951; Fernandez Diaz et al., 1964). This protein exists in three forms (A_3, A_2, and A_1), which is due to different amounts of phosphate, 0, 1, and 2 moieties, respectively (Pearlman, 1952). Two other types of ovalbumin have been reported. One is plakalbumin (Linderstrom-Lang and Ottesen, 1947; Ottesen, 1958) which results from the cleavage of a heptapeptide from ovalbumin. The other is a stable product, S-ovalbumin (Smith, 1964).

The properties of ovomucin have been extensively investigated (Osuga and Feeney, 1968; Donovan et al., 1970; Robinson and Monsey, 1971). One of the earliest characteristic properties asso-ciated with ovomucin fractions was the viral antihemaglutination activity (Gottschalk and Lind, 1959). This glycoprotein is apparent-ly responsible for the gel-like properties of egg white, and has been implicated in its aging properties (Feeney and Allison, 1969).

TABLE I

Physical Properties of Egg-White Proteins[a]

Protein	Amount in egg white (%)	pI	Mol wt (gm)	$s_{20,w}$	$D_{20,w} \times 10^7$ (cm² sec⁻¹)	$\bar{V}$ (cm³/gm)	$E^{1\%}_\lambda$
Ovalbumin	54	4.5	46,000	3.27	7.67	0.750	$E^{1\%}_{280} = 7.50$
Ovotransferrin	12	6.05	76,600	5.05	5.72(Fe)	0.732	$E^{1\%}_{280} = 11.6$
Ovomucoid	11	4.1	28,000	2.62	7.7	0.685	$E^{1\%}_{280} = 4.55$
Lysozyme	3.4	10.7	14,300	1.91	11.2	0.703	$E^{1\%}_{280} = 26.35$
Ovomucin[b]	3.5	4.5–5.0	110,000 ± 20,000	6.4(10%) 2.9(5%) 1.4(85%)	nd	nd	$E^{1\%}_{277.5} = 9.3$
Ovoinhibitor	1.5	5.1	49,000 44,000	—	nd	0.693	$E^{1\%}_{278} = 7.4$
Ovomacroglobulin	0.5	4.5	900,000 760,000	15.1	1.98	0.745	
Ovoglycoprotein	1.0	3.9	24,400	2.47	nd	nd	$E^{1\%}_{280} = 3.8$
Ovoflavoprotein	0.8	4.0	32,000	2.76	6.4	0.70	$E^{1\%}_{280} = 15.3^c$
Avidin	0.05	10	68,300	4.55	5.98	0.73^d	$E^{1\%}_{280} = 15.7$

[a] Adapted from Feeney and Allison (1969), Table 2-2.

[b] Donovan et al. (1970) $s_{20,w}$ and molecular weight by osmotic pressure were measured in 6 M guanidine·HCl with 0.2 M mercaptoethanol.

[c] D. T. Osuga and R. E. Feeney, unpublished data.

[d] Green (1963d).

42

Ovomacroglobulin was reported the most immunogenic minor constituent present in egg white, and also had the greatest antigenic cross-reactivity among various avian species (Miller and Feeney, 1964). This protein was first isolated and characterized by Miller and Feeney (1966). Recently, Donovan et al. (1969) demonstrated the presence of subunit structure.

Ovoglycoprotein, another minor constituent, is unusual for egg-white proteins in that it has not been reported to possess any particular characteristic property (Ketterer, 1962, 1965).

The numerous minor avian egg-white constituents have been recently reviewed by Baker (1968) and Feeney and Allison (1969). Since these comprehensive reviews, the enzymic properties of β-N-acetylglucosaminidase and of catalase have been described by Donovan and Hansen (1971a,b) and by Ball and Cotterill (1971a, b), respectively, and Baker (1970) has reviewed genetic polymorphism in egg-white proteins.

B. COMPARATIVE BIOCHEMISTRY

Comparative biochemistry of avian egg-white proteins from various species and their homologous and analogous relationships to proteins from milk and blood, were extensively discussed and reviewed by Feeney and Allison (1969). Therefore, in this section only a brief summary of the comparative biochemistry of the selected egg-white proteins (Table I, italic, and Table II) will be presented.

Ovotransferrins from various avian egg whites have a number of characteristically similar properties, e.g., those relating to binding metal ions, existence in multiple molecular forms, absorption spectra, temperature stability, size ($s_{20,w}$), and electron spin resonance spectra. However, notable differences do exist, especially in electrophoretic mobilities, composition, and amounts present in various avian egg whites (Feeney and Allison, 1969).

Protein inhibitors of proteolytic enzymes have been reported in chicken egg white. Papain and ficin were reported to be inhibited by a papain inhibitor (Fossum and Whitaker, 1968). Ovoinhibitor inhibits a number of enzymes, whereas chicken ovomucoid is specific for one enzyme (Table III). Recently, Liu et al. (1971)

TABLE II
Amino Acid Composition of Egg-White Proteins

	Avidin[a] (residues per subunit)	Ovomucoid[b] (residues per 28,000 gm)	Ovoinhibitor[c] (residues per 49,000 gm)	Ovotransferrin[d] (residues per 76,000 gm)	Ovoflavoprotein[e] (residues per 32,000 gm)	Lysozyme[f] (residues per 14,307 gm)
Alanine	5	11.7	20.1	52	13.9	12
Arginine	8	6.3	20.5	33	5.6	11
Aspartic acid	15	31.9	47.3	79	20.0	8(13)[g]
Cystine/2	2	17.5	34.7	22	15.9	8
Glutamic acid	10	14.9	40.7	69	36.4	2(3)[g]
Glycine	11	16.1	32.3	58	8.3	12
Histidine	1	4.3	12.9	13	9.2	1
Isoleucine	8	3.2	17.3	24	7.1	6
Leucine	7	12.2	22.4	48	14.8	8
Lysine	9	13.6	24.2	62	17.2	6
Methionine	2	1.9	3.6	11	8.2	2
Phenylalanine	7	5.3	6.4	25	7.0	3
Proline	2	7.7	17.2	31	9.7	2

Serine	9	12.5	26.0	42	28.8	10
Threonine	21	14.6	28.0	35	7.7	7
Tryptophan	4	0	1.0	18	8.8	6
Tyrosine	1	6.7	15.1	20	9.5	3
Valine	7	16.0	25.9	44	5.7	6
Sialic acid	0[h]	0.3		0[l]	0.5[l]	
Hexose		12–16.5[j]	5–10[k]		14%	
Mannose	5[j]	10–13.4[j]		4[m]	Present	
Galactose	4[l]	0.8–6.3[j]			Present	
Glucosamine	0	14.8–27.7[j]	7–15[k]	6[m]	Present	
Galactosamine		0	0			
N-Terminal	Alanine[n]	Alanine[n]	Alanine[n]	Alanine[n]	Serine and glycine[o]	Lysine
C-Terminal	Glutamic acid	Glutamic acid				Leucine

[a] DeLange (1970); DeLange and Huang (1971).
[b] Osuga and Feeney (1968).
[c] Calculated from Liu et al. (1971).
[d] Calculated from Williams (1962).
[e] Farrell et al. (1969).
[f] Canfield (1963).
[g] Value in parenthesis are amides.
[h] Green (1963b).
[i] Feeney et al. (1960).
[j] Calculated from Beeley (1971).
[k] Davis et al. (1969).
[l] Huang and DeLange (1971).
[m] Phillips and Azari (1971).
[n] Fraenkel-Conrat and Porter (1952).
[o] Two C-terminal reported by Phillips et al. (1969).

described the properties of five ovoinhibitors (chicken, turkey, duck, penguin, and quail). These combine in a ratio of 2 moles of trypsin and 2 moles of α-chymotrypsin per mole of inhibitor (48,000 gm). Penguin ovoinhibitor was unusual in that it did not inhibit α-chymotrypsin, but all the ovoinhibitors from various species required arginine for trypsin inhibition (to be discussed later in Section V). Arginine requirement was in contrast to the trypsin inhibitory activity of the ovomucoids from 12 avian species, in which lysine residue was involved in inhibition in 11 of the 12 (Stevens and Feeney, 1963; Haynes *et al.*, 1967; Feeney, 1971b). Only chicken ovomucoid had arginine as the essential residue. The wide variation in specificity of some of the inhibitors in avian egg white is summarized in Table III. A notable general characteristic of the inhibitors was that all α-chymotrypsin inhibitors were also subtilisin inhibitors. Of all the avian egg-white inhibitors investigated in our laboratory, only quail ovomucoid was a good inhibitor of human trypsin (Feeney *et al.*, 1969). The recent important observations by Gertler and Feinstein (1971) concerning the inhibition of porcine elastase by turkey ovomucoid and chicken ovoinhibitor are footnoted in Table III.

Feeney and Allison (1969), Feeney (1971b), and Lin and Feeney (1972) reviewed some of the various aspects of ovomucoids from several avian species. In general, they have similar molecular sizes, acidic isoelectric points, and are composed of multiple molecular forms. However, not only do they vary in composition, they also differ in inhibitory specificities.

Lysozyme is the most thoroughly investigated egg-white protein. Since determination of the amino acid sequence of chicken egg-white lysozyme in 1963 (Canfield, 1963; Jollès *et al.*, 1963), a number of other avian egg-white lysozymes have had their sequence determined—turkey (La Rue and Speck, 1970); duck (Hermann and Jollès, 1970; Hermann *et al.*, 1971); guinea hen (Jollès *et al.*, 1972) and Japanese quail (Kaneda *et al.*, 1969). Recently Canfield *et al.* (1971) reviewed some of the different characteristics of goose and chicken egg-white lysozymes. Feeney and Allison (1969) summarized the earlier work on the differences among chicken, duck, and goose egg-white lysozyme. Prager and Wilson (1971a) isolated and investigated three lysozymes from duck egg white. They com-

TABLE III
Inhibition of Five Proteinases by Ovomucoids and Ovoinhibitors[a]

	Enzymes inhibited[b]				
	Human trypsin	Bovine trypsin	Bovine α-chymotrypsin	Subtilisin	Fungal proteinase[c]
Ovomucoids					
Chicken	−	+++	−	−	−
Quail	++	+++	−	−	−
Cassowary	−	++	−	−	−
Ostrich	−	+	−	−	−
Emu	−	++	+	+	−
Rhea	−	++	+	+	−
Pheasant[d]	−	−	++++	+++	−
Duck	−	++++	++++	+++	−
Turkey[e]	−	++++	++++	++	−
Tinamou	−	+	++++	++	−
Penguin	−	+	++	++++	−
Ovoinhibitors					
Chicken[e]	−	++++	++++	++++	++++
Quail	?	++++	++++	++++	++++
Turkey	?	++++	++++	++++	++++
Penguin	?	++++	−	++++	++++

[a]From Feeney (1971b), Table 3.
[b]Enzymatic activity determined by the casein digestion assay. The degree of inhibition is indicated as (−) for extremely weak or inactive ($K_{diss} < 10^{-5}$ M) and +, ++, +++, and ++++, for varying degrees, progressing from weak ($K_{diss} \sim 10^{-5}$ M) to strong ($K_{diss} \sim > 10^{-9}$ M).
[c]Alkaline proteinase from *Aspergillus oryzae.*
[d]Golden pheasant.
[e]Gertler and Feinstein (1971) reported that elastase was inhibited by turkey ovomucoid and chicken ovoinhibitor; elastase competed with α-chymotrypsin and fungal proteinase (from *A. sojae*) for ovomucoid and ovoinhibitor, respectively.

pared their results from amino acid analysis with previously published results, and reported that they could not find a histidine containing lysozyme as previously reported by Jollès *et al.* (1965). Polymorphism in lysozymes was shown to exist in ducks (Prager and Wilson, 1971a), quails (Baker and Manwell, 1967), black swan (Arnheim and Steller, 1970), and geese (Arnheim and Steller, 1970).

The black swan egg-white lysozymes had a very interesting immunological cross-reaction (Arnheim and Steller, 1970). One lysozyme would react with chicken egg-white lysozyme and the second with goose egg-white lysozyme. Immunological analyses of 16 galliforms were reported by Arnheim and Wilson (1967). The interpretations of their technique were verified by amino acid analysis of egg-white lysozymes from quail and ring-necked pheasant (Arnheim *et al.*, 1969), and by comparing their results with those obtained with lysozymes of known amino acid composition (Prager and Wilson, 1971b). The method was then used to indicate the percentage of cross-reaction of various lysozymes (Prager and Wilson, 1971c). In their study, no cross-reaction occurred between egg-white lysozyme and human lysozyme or with α-lactalbumin. Fauré and Jollès (1970) reported on the low antigenicity and structural similarities among human milk lysozyme, α-lactalbumin, and goose egg-white lysozyme compared to those among chicken, guinea hen, and duck egg-white lysozymes.

There are only a few reports on the comparative aspects of avidin and ovoflavoprotein. The amounts of these two proteins in various avian egg whites were tabulated by Feeney and Allison (1969). The degree of yellow color in chicken egg white was shown by Bain and Deutsch (1948) to be dependent upon the diet. Rhodes *et al.* (1959) demonstrated that the binding capacity of chicken egg white remained unchanged due to the effect of fluctuating the flavin content of the diet, nor could they increase the riboflavin content in duck egg whites from its normal very low level. Riboflavin administered orally or by injection did not increase the flavin content in penguin egg white (Feeney *et al.*, 1968) nor in duck or goose egg white (Rhodes *et al.*, 1960a).

III. Avidin—The Principal Toxic Constituent

A. HISTORY AND TOXIC EFFECTS

Avidin is a protein responsible for a syndrome produced by the presence of egg white in the diet of rats (Boas, 1924). In a further study, Boas (1927) described the effects produced when desiccated egg white was fed. Briefly, the following sequence of events occurred: dermatitis, baldness, nervous disorder (kangaroo-like posture and movement of the front feet), and death.

Parsons and Kelly (1933a, b) substantiated the results obtained by Boas. They demonstrated the presence of the toxic factor in egg whites of fresh eggs, stored eggs, and dried eggs, and in Chinese fermented dried egg white (dried egg white produced in China). The toxic effects were destroyed by heating the material at 80°C for 5 minutes, except for the Chinese fermented dried egg white which required 18 times longer heat treatment. The material in egg white was therefore called the "Chinese dried egg white injury factor." They also reported the detoxification effect of HCl and peptic hydrolysis, and that the toxic factor was a protein which precipitated in saturated ammonium sulfate.

The microbiological assay of biotin was one of the more important developments which led to the identification of the cause of egg-white injury (Snell et al., 1940). Subsequently the assay was modified to study the egg-white toxic factor, and ultimately led to the concentration of that factor (Eakin et al., 1940a, 1941; Woolley and Longsworth, 1942). Pennington et al. (1942) crystallized avidin from the purified avidin fraction from egg white. Formation of a complex between avidin and biotin was shown both in vivo and in vitro in 1940. Parsons et al. (1940) were able to cure egg-white injury in rats by feeding them heated feces from rats fed a diet of raw egg white. Unheated feces from the same source had no curative effect. György and Rose (1941) also noted that a complex existed in the feces. Eakin et al. (1940a) mixed their concentrated sample of egg-white toxic factor with biotin and demonstrated the absence of free biotin by the microbiological assay system of Snell et al. (1940). No biotin was released when the sample was dialyzed in the pH range of 2–10.5, but upon steam heating, biotin was released and detected in the dialysate. Eakin et al. (1940b) showed that chicks on a ration of raw egg white, and rich in biotin (0.67 μg/gm of diet) compared to the control group (0.39 μg/gm of diet), had less biotin in their tissues. Thus it became evident that avidin and biotin formed a stable complex which could not be absorbed in the intestinal tract, and which was excreted in the feces.

Symptoms of egg-white injury occur in the presence of avidin or with a deficiency of biotin in the diet. The effect has been produced by a raw egg-white diet, and corrected by injection of biotin, not only in rats and chicks, but also in hamsters (Rauch and Nutting, 1958), man (Sydenstricker *et al.*, 1942), and pigs (Cunha *et al.*, 1946). György (1954) listed a number of vertebrates which have been affected by egg-white injury (dogs, piglets, turkeys, cows, fish, and monkeys).

Peters (1967) has described, in rats, a fulminating effect of raw egg white which could be corrected by a diet of heat-denatured egg white, but not by a biotin supplement. The effect in this case appeared unlike egg-white injury resulting from biotin deficiency. The diet, plus administration of caffeine and benzylpenicillin, resulted in the death of the rat. No deaths were reported in the absence of caffeine, whereas with caffeine (185 mg/kg of rat), death usually occurred within a week. Death could not be prevented by administration of 200 μg biotin (Peters and Boyd, 1966). Benzylpenicillin in the normal diet of rats produced no ill effects, but the combination of the drug and raw egg white resulted in a skin reaction (Boyd and Sargeant, 1962). Injection of subcutaneous biotin permitted the animal to survive 2 weeks and prevented the appearance of dermatitis, but did not inhibit the neurological signs. Identity of the factor or factors responsible for these effects of raw egg white remains unknown.

B. ISOLATION AND ASSAY

Carboxymethyl cellulose (CM-cellulose) has been used successfully in the purification of avidin from egg white in large quantities (Rhodes *et al.*, 1958). Avidin prepared by this technique, and by alternate methods (see below) was free of any complex with nucleic acid or acidic glycoproteins. Melamed and Green (1963), using three successive CM-cellulose chromatographies and then Amberlite CG-50, obtained preparations containing as much as 13.8 units/mg avidin. A unit of activity of avidin is the amount of avidin required for inactivating 1 μg of biotin. The two avidin fractions obtained from Amberlite CG-50 varied only in amino acid composition. Using a similar technique of isolation, Green and associates have isolated avidin with a very high binding capacity (15.1 units/mg avidin) (Green, 1970a), and have crystallized avidin in three forms (Green and Toms, 1970). The crystals were in the form of square plates, rather thick plates, and needlelike shapes. The latter type crystal has recently been used for preliminary crystallographic investigations (Green and Joynson, 1970).

Affinity chromatography of avidin has been reported by McCormick (1965) and Cuatrecasas and Wilchek (1968). The methods they used were based upon previous reports by Wright *et al.* (1950) and Green (1963c) that both biocytin (ε-N-biotinyl-L-lysine) and biotin formed strong complexes with avidin, and that the carboxyl group of biotin was not essential for complex formation. McCormick (1965) esterified the carboxyl group of biotin to cellulose and applied a sample of commercial avidin. He attained a 10-fold purification of the sample which resulted in a product with 12 units/mg avidin. The elution of the major avidin peak was effected by lowering the ionic strength. Cuatrecasas and Wilchek (1968) coupled the amino group of biocytin to Sepharose. Recovery of binding activity from the application of crude egg white was 90% of the total biotin-binding activity and a 4000-fold purification of avidin. The sample was eluted with a reversible denaturing reagent, 6 M guanidine·HCl, at pH 1.5. This resulted in a product with 14 units/mg of avidin activity.

The sensitive microbiological assay techniques for avidin or biotin were based on the growth of a strain of *Saccharomyces cerevisiae* (Snell *et al.*, 1940). By this method, 0.00002–0.001 μg of biotin could be quantitated. Green (1962), using several spectrophotometric methods for assaying avidin, reported that at 233 nm there was a 25% increase in absorbancy, due to the formation of a complex between avidin and biotin. The spectral shift was the basis for two types of assay techniques, a difference spectrum and a titration technique (Green, 1963c). Green (1965) also introduced another spectrophotometric procedure using an azo dye, 4-hydroxyazobenzene-2'-carboxylic acid. The addition of the dye to an excess of avidin caused an increase in extinction, at 500 nm, from 600 to 34,500, in addition to a drastic decrease at 348 nm. The absorption changes were reversed by the addition of biotin. The sensitivity of this technique is approximately 25 units/ml of avidin. Another widely used assay system utilizes radioactive biotin (Green, 1963a). This is a rapid and simple method in which the complex between ^{14}C-biotin and avidin is absorbed on CM-cellulose, and the unabsorbed ^{14}C-biotin determined. This procedure has a higher sensitivity but less accuracy than the spectrophotometric methods described above. Wei and Wright (1964) used ^{14}C-biotin and separated the complex from excess ^{14}C-biotin on a column of Sephadex G-25. Korenman and O'Malley (1967) using ^{14}C-biotin, absorbed the complex on bentonite. Sensitivity was about 0.1 μg/ml avidin. Immunoassays have been used by O'Malley and Korenman (1967). Refined step-by-step assay procedures have recently been described (Green, 1970b; Wei, 1970; Korenman and O'Malley, 1970).

C. GENERAL PROPERTIES

Avidin is a basic glycoprotein, has a molecular weight of approximately 70,000 gm (Table I), is composed of 4 polypeptide subunits (Green, 1964b), and has an isoelectric point at pH 10 (Woolley and Longsworth, 1942). Green and Toms (1970) and DeLange (1970) found 129 amino acid residues per subunit (Table II). DeLange and Huang (1971) recently completed the amino acid sequence of avidin by analysis of cyanogen bromide and tryptic fragments (DeLange, 1970; Huang and DeLange, 1971). Their sequence work indicated the presence of 13 amide groups and 128 amino acid residues, whereas amino acid analysis indicated 16 and 129, respectively. The complete sequence of the protein subunit indicates that there is no sequence similarity between avidin and lysozyme, as previously suggested by Green (1968).

Although heterogeneity of avidin has been reported (Fraenkel-Conrat *et al.*, 1952a; Green, 1963b), DeLange and Huang (1971) identified only one sequence heterogeneity; residue number 34 was ½ isoleucine and ½ threonine. Thus, Table II for avidin should indicate that there are 20½ threonines and 7½ isoleucines and that half of the avidin subunits contain threonine and the other half isoleucine at residue number 34. Carbohydrate analysis of the only tryptic peptide found by Huang and DeLange (1971) indicated that there were four residues of glucosamine and five residues of mannose present in an avidin subunit.

Avidin binds four biotins, one per subunit (Green, 1964b), to form a strongly associated complex with a dissociation constant of $10^{-5}\,M$ and a free energy change of 20 kcal/mole of biotin bound (Green, 1963a). The rate of formation is $7 \times 10^7\,M^{-1}\,sec^{-1}$, and the reverse rate is $9 \times 10^{-8}\,M^{-1}\,sec^{-1}$. Because the rate of formation is so rapid, Green (1963a) concluded that the reaction rate is diffusion-controlled. Important features of biotin for binding to avidin appear to be the ureido ring and the aliphatic chain portion. The carboxyl and the thioether groups appear to be unnecessary for complex formation.

Studies of the interaction between avidin and biotin by fluorescence polarization of the dinitrophenylhydrazide of biotin indicated that the four binding sites of the tetramer were independent and combined in a random fashion (Green, 1964a). This binding did not result in any gross change in the structure of avidin, as the optical rotation and optical rotatory dispersion did not change significantly (Green, 1962; Pritchard *et al.*, 1966; Green and Melamed, 1966). Polarization of fluorescence of avidin labeled with a 1-dimethylaminonapthalene-5-sulfonyl group also revealed only a slight change when the complex was formed (Green, 1963d). The binding force in biotin binding is considered to be of hydrophobic nature. This view is supported by the lack of entropy change during complex formation (Green, 1966). Studies of the oxidation of tryptophan of avidin by N-bromosuccinimide indicated that each molecule of biotin protects four tryptophan residues of the avidin from oxidation by the reagent, and that each subunit reacts independently of each other (Green, 1962, 1963a,c; Green and Ross, 1968). The oxidation of an average of one tryptophan per subunit did not cause a decrease in binding activity, but the loss of two caused approximately 90% loss. The spectral shift due to the binding was interpreted to reflect a change in the environment of the tryptophan residue from partially aqueous to nonpolar.

Formation of an avidin–biotin complex results in an unusually stable compound which is resistant to denaturation and proteolysis (György and Rose, 1943). The presence of various ions interferes with complex formation and the release of biotin from the complex (Pai and Lichstein, 1964). Boiling the complex for 10 and 60 minutes released 88 and 99% of the biotin, respectively. The ionic strength of the medium is important for the stability of the complex (Wei and Wright, 1964). Although avidin is quite labile to steaming at 100°C, little (10%) or no biotin is released after the complex has been steamed 15 minutes in 0.2 M ammonium carbonate. Complete dissociation can be attained by autoclaving at 120°C for 15 minutes. Pritchard et al. (1966) demonstrated that avidin was irreversibly denatured at temperatures greater than 70°C, but that the complex remained stable until 100°C. The temperatures for irreversible denaturation of avidin and its biotin complex were 85° and 132°C, respectively. The corresponding enthalpies of denaturation were 290 and 1000 kcal/mole, respectively (Donovan and Ross, 1972).

Fraenkel-Conrat et al. (1952b) concluded that the binding site of avidin does not contain a reactive amino, phenolic, imidazole, carboxyl, or disulfide group. Loss of avidin activity was noted in the presence of trace metals, especially iron. The complex was also sensitive to light and metal ions (Fraenkel-Conrat et al., 1952a). Avidin is quite stable in 8 M urea (Fraenkel-Conrat et al., 1952a), but not in 6 M guanidine·HCl (Green, 1963d). The denaturating effect of 6 M guanidine·HCl can be reversed by a 10-fold dilution, and reversible denaturation also occurs below pH 2. Fluorescence-polarization experiments reveal that avidin does not dissociate into subunits in 3 M guanidine·HCl, and that the complex does not dissociate in 6 M guanidine·HCl (Green, 1963d).

Crosslinking of avidin molecules with a bifunctional biotin amide, bisbiotinylpolymethylenediamine, has been used to determine the spatial relationships of the biotin binding groups in the subunits (Green, 1967; Green et al., 1971). A series of the bifunctional reagents containing methylene groups ranging from 9 to 25 was used. When there were less than 12 methylene groups, only 1 of the 2 biotins in the bifunctional reagent was bound. With greater distance between the two biotins, with 12, 13, or 14 methylene groups, some polymers were formed; but these were reported to be very weak and could easily be displaced by a weak-binding analog of biotin. Lengths from 15 to 22 groups formed stable complexes, and polymers were detected. These were probably the result of

intermolecular binding. But those bifunctional reagents with greater than 22 groups did not form polymers, indicating a binding
of 2 subunits within the avidin molecule. Green and associates thus
concluded that the avidin molecules were arranged with 222 symmetry, and that the binding sites were grouped in 2 pairs at opposite
ends with a dimension of 55 Å × 55 Å × 41 Å. The symmetry and
dimensions agree well with the X-ray crystallographic studies by
Green and Joynson (1970).

IV. Lysozyme—The Bacteriolytic Agent in Egg White

A. History

Egg white was early observed by microscopic analysis to lyse
some organisms (Laschtschenko, 1909). In 1922, Fleming described
the lytic substance from egg white which lyses micrococcus cells.
He named this enzyme lysozyme, and the air micrococcus which
he found, *Micrococcus lysodeikticus.*

Lysozyme was first reported to be crystallized by Abraham and
Robinson (1937). Alderton and Fevold (1946) described a high-
yielding, simple, and direct method of crystallization from egg
white. The easy availability of the crystalline form of the enzyme,
and its low molecular weight, have contributed to its use in a series
of well-known fundamental investigations in protein and enzyme
chemistry: (1) hypothesis that the conformation of a molecule is
dictated by its primary structure (Isemura *et al.,* 1961); (2) the
direction of peptide chain synthesis is from the NH_2-terminal
toward the COOH-terminal end (Canfield and Anfinsen, 1963);
(3) the first enzyme and the third protein to have its tertiary structure determined by X-ray crystallography (Blake *et al.,* 1965); (4)
the first enzyme in which a reasonable reaction mechanism was
proposed entirely by crystalline structure analysis (Blake *et al.,*
1967).

The early investigations were reviewed by Thompson (1940).
More recent reviews are by Salton (1964), Jollès (1964), Phillips
(1967), Raftery and Dahlquist (1969), Feeney and Allison (1969),
and Chipman and Sharon (1969).

B. GENERAL PHYSICAL, CHEMICAL, AND BIOCHEMICAL PROPERTIES

The physical properties and chemical composition of lysozyme are tabulated in Tables I and II respectively. Although its molecular size is small (14,307 gm), the enzyme predominantly exists as a dimer between pH 5 and 9 (Sophianopoulous and Van Holde, 1964). The amino acid sequence was reported independently by two laboratories (Canfield, 1963; Jollès *et al.*, 1963).

This enzyme was reported to be extremely stable in acid to alkaline pH, but less stable in alkali, and inactivated in the presence of copper. It was stable upon heating at pH 4.5 and 100°C for 1–2 minutes. Even after 6 years, much of the enzymic activity remained at pH 3.4–9.1, at room temperature and exposed to laboratory lighting (Feeney *et al.*, 1956).

Lysozyme will enzymically cleave bacterial cell walls and chitin. It cleaves specifically at the β-(1–4) glycosidic linkages between polymers of N-acetylglucosamine and N-acetylmuramic acid. Thus the enzyme (EC 3.2.1.17; mucopeptide N-acetylmuramylhydrolase) has been called lysozyme, mucopeptide glucohydrolase, and muramidase. A *trans*-glycosylation reaction has also been described for lysozyme (Chipman and Sharon, 1969). The enzymic activity is inhibited by a number of N-acetylhexosamines (Blake *et al.*, 1967).

The active site of lysozyme contains specific amino acid residues (3 aspartyl, 3 tryptophanyl, and 1 glutamyl) which interact with the carbohydrate polymer to cause cleavage. Chipman and Sharon (1969) and Spande *et al.* (1970) have recently reviewed the chemical and crystallographic investigations on lysozyme.

Light (1951) reported that lysozyme was toxic, as it was one of the substances present in closed-loop intestinal obstruction. This was refuted by Lobstein (1961), who demonstrated that intravenous injection of lysozyme (55 mg lysozyme/kg anmal) was nontoxic to dogs. Miller and Campbell (1950) reported that lysozyme produced a positive intradermal response more frequently than did ovalbumin, ovomucin, or ovomucoid. Vaughan and Kabat (1954) observed that lysozyme produced a positive response in both control and sensitized sites. Bleumink and Young (1969, 1971) also obtained a positive skin test with lysozyme, but much less than that with the other egg-white proteins (0.6% of that produced by ovomucoid). Thus, they concluded that lysozyme produced a nonspecific positive reaction.

V. Ovomucoid and Ovoinhibitor

A. HISTORY

Ovomucoid was first isolated and named in 1894 by Morner and an antitrypsin property was reported in egg white by Delezene and Pozerski in 1904 and by Hedin in 1907. However, it was not until 40 years later that Lineweaver and Murray (1947) demonstrated that ovomucoid was responsible for the antitrypsin property in egg white.

Matsushima (1958a, b) described a second inhibitor present in egg white and named it ovoinhibitor. This protein not only inhibited bovine trypsin, but also bacterial proteinase from *Baccillus subtilis* var. *biotecus* and fungal proteinase from an unidentified species of *Aspergillus*. Ovoinhibitor was then found to inhibit bovine chymotrypsin and a fungal proteinase from *A. oryzae* (Rhodes *et al.*, 1960b). Feeney *et al.* (1963) found that ovoinhibitor was a contaminate present in most chicken ovomucoid preparations, and that the inhibitory activity against chymotrypsin reported for chicken ovomucoid was due to the presence of the ovoinhibitor.

Numerous reviews on ovomucoid and ovoinhibitor have been published. Earlier reviews were by Meyer (1945), Fevold (1951), Laskowski and Laskowski (1954), and Warner (1954); more recent reviews were by Melamed (1966), Vogel *et al.* (1969), Feeney and Allison (1969), Kassell (1970), Feeney (1971a, b), and Lin and Feeney (1972).

B. GENERAL PHYSICAL, CHEMICAL, AND BIOCHEMICAL PROPERTIES

The general physical and chemical properties of ovomucoid and ovoinhibitor are listed in Tables I and II.

Ovomucoid and ovoinhibitor are among the larger (28,000 and 49,000 gm, respectively) of the naturally occurring protein inhibitors (Liener and Kakade, 1969; Feeney and Allison, 1969). These two inhibitors exist in multiple molecular forms, but do not contain subunits. Molecular heterogeneity of ovomucoid was first reported by Longsworth et al. (1940), and has not yet been completely resolved. However, Beeley (1971) recently reported on the complete separation and analysis of the different multiple molecular forms. He substantiated earlier implications that the gross differences were due to the carbohydrate content (Beeley and Jevons, 1965; Feeney et al., 1967) and the presence of minor variations in amino acid composition of the various forms (Feeney et al., 1967). Tomimatsu et al. (1966) showed that ovoinhibitor was composed of multiple molecular forms, and Davis et al. (1969) separated and characterized the various forms. The gross differences were also attributed to the variation in carbohydrate content.

Ovomucoid (Lineweaver and Murray, 1947) and ovoinhibitor (Matsushima, 1958a, b) were shown to be relatively stable proteins. Ovomucoid retained more than 90% of its activity in 9 M urea at pH 4 after incubation for 18 hours at 25°C, and between the pH range of 3–7 for 30 minutes at 80°C. Ovoinhibitor was stable in acidic solutions, with approximately 95% of its activity being retained at pH 3 and 5 when incubated for 15 minutes at 90°C. Both inhibitors were somewhat labile at alkaline pH. Heating ovomucoid at pH 9 and 80°C for 30 minutes resulted in 94% loss of activity (Stevens and Feeney, 1963). Ovoinhibitor lost all its activity in 0.1 N NaOH at 40°C for 3 hours, and in 15 minutes at pH 7 and 9 at 90°C. Matsushima (1958a) reported it to be stable in 0.01 N NaOH at 23°C for 24 hours.

Chemical modification of the amino groups in ovomucoid caused no loss of activity (Stevens and Feeney, 1963), but arginine was necessary for activity (Ozawa and Laskowski, 1966; Liu et al., 1968). Arginine was also shown to be necessary for the activity of ovoinhibitor (Liu et al., 1971).

The mechanism by which ovomucoid inhibits trypsin was early suggested to involve a highly associated enzyme–substrate complex in which the substrate is hydrolyzed only very slowly by the enzyme (Sri et al., 1954). Chemical modifications of side-chain residues have revealed that specific residues (lysines in ovomucoids other than in chicken) are usually essential for inhibitory activity (Haynes *et al.*, 1967; Feeney, 1971a). Precise chemical kinetics and identifications of bonds hydrolyzed in complexes have proven that the peptide bond of a particular arginine may be attacked (Ozawa and Laskowski, 1966; Laskowski *et al.*, 1971). According to these investigators, the main driving force for the formation of the highly associated enzyme-inhibitor complex is the catalytic action of the enzyme on the inhibitor, i.e., the formation of a covalent bond by the acylation of the serine in the enzyme by the arginyl carboxyl of the inhibitor. However, other studies indicate that the main strength of the interaction may not be due to covalent bonds, but rather to the forces commonly encountered in other protein–protein complexes, such as antigen–antibody complexes. According to this interpretation, the enzyme recognizes the inhibitor as a substrate and forms a specific complex, but the main forces are noncovalent ones, such as hydrogen bonds and van der Waals forces (Feeney, 1971a). In support of this idea, several ovomucoids were shown to form strongly associated complexes with catalytically inert derivatives of trypsin or chymotrypsin (Feinstein and Feeney, 1966). Whether covalent bond formation is only secondary rather than of primary importance may not be known until X-ray analyses of the complexes are made.

Chicken ovomucoid was for a long time accepted as an inhibitor of human trypsin as well as of bovine trypsin. This apparently was still the case even after a short note in 1962 (Buck *et al.*, 1962) stated it was a poor inhibitor of human trypsin! It was finally proven that neither chicken ovomucoid nor chicken ovoinhibitor have detectable activity against human trypsin (Feeney *et al.*, 1969). This lack of activity is in direct agreement with results of human feeding tests. Scudamore *et al.* (1949) reported that there was no effect upon nitrogen retention by human subjects from feeding powdered commercial egg white, raw or heated, as a supplemental source of dietary protein with chemically isolated ovomucoid. When young rats were fed ovomucoid at levels of 2.5% in a casein diet, Klose *et al.* (1950) observed no effects on growth or protein efficiency.

The different inhibitory specificities of ovomucoids against human and bovine trypsins (Table III) illustrate the necessity for care in extrapolating data from one species to another. The observation (Gertler and Feinstein, 1971) that ovoinhibitor inhibits nonhuman elastase must also be considered in the same light.

The clinical, allergenic, and laboratory effects of egg-white proteins, particularly ovomucoid, have been discussed and reviewed in several recent articles. Ankier (1969) reported that ovomucoid produced an anaphylactoid response in rats, and that many of the egg-white proteins were anaphylactic antigens. Vogel *et al.* (1969), in reviewing experimental effects of ovomucoid, reported that it influences vascular permeability, stimulates pancreatic secretion, causes local inflammation and anaphylactic shock, and inhibits plasma kallikrein. Egg white was also stated to inhibit reversibly human urine kallikrein. Bleumink and Young (1969, 1971) reviewed the allergenic effects of egg-white proteins and ovomucoid. Ovomucoid was considered the major factor in egg white responsible for the positive skin reactivity induced by intracutaneous injection into atopic individuals. Ovoinhibitor, ovoflavoprotein, ovalbumin, and lysozyme also produced positive skin reactions, but the effects were much less than that from ovomucoid.

VI. Ovotransferrin

A. History

Osborne and Campbell (1900) isolated from egg white a protein which precipitated with ovalbumin during ammonium sulfate fractionation. They called it conalbumin. Ovotransferrin is the current name which is widely accepted because of its close homology with blood serum transferrin (Feeney and Allison, 1969).

Schade and Caroline (1944) found that the inhibitory effects of raw egg white on the growth of several microorganisms could be overcome by the addition of excess iron. This bacteria-inhibiting protein in the egg white was due to the presence of ovotransferrin (Alderton *et al.*, 1946). The copper-binding capacity in egg white was also associated with ovotransferrin (Fraenkel-Conrat and Feeney, 1950). Warner and Weber (1951) first crystallized iron-ovotransferrin.

Ovotransferrin has been reviewed by Feeney and Komatsu (1966) and Feeney and Allison (1969).

B. GENERAL PHYSICAL, CHEMICAL, AND BIOCHEMICAL PROPERTIES

The principal distinctive feature of ovotransferrin is the binding with 2 atoms of iron per mole of protein, and the resulting salmon-pink color (Schade *et al.*, 1949) with an absorption maximum at 465 nm. Copper also complexes with the protein to produce a yellow color (Fraenkel-Conrat and Feeney, 1950) with an absorption maximum at 440 nm. The binding ratio was 2 atoms of metal at 2 specific binding sites per mole of protein. The relative strengths of these complexes were $Fe^{3+} > Cu^{2+} > Zn^{2+}$ (Fraenkel-Conrat and Feeney, 1950; Warner and Weber, 1953). More recently the displacement studies of Tan and Woodworth (1969) indicated the following relative stabilities:

$$Fe^{3+} > Cr^{3+}, Cu^{2+} > Mn^{2+}, Co^{2+}, Cd^{2+} > Zn^{2+} > Ni^{2+}$$

The metal-binding site in ovotransferrin appears to involve several specific amino acid residues (Fraenkel-Conrat and Feeney, 1950). The bicarbonate ion has also been reported to be an important factor in producing a colored iron-ovotransferrin (Warner and Weber, 1953). Aisen *et al.* (1967) reported that the complex can be formed in the absence of bicarbonate, and that the bicarbonate ion can be replaced by a reagent with two or more carboxyl groups to form a colored complex of iron-transferrin. However, Price and Gibson (1972) reported that the bicarbonate ion is necessary for the detection of iron-transferrin complexes by electron paramagnetic resonance. Carboxyl groups, tyrosines, histidines, and tryptophans have, at various times, been implicated as binding ligands for iron in transferrins. Wishnia *et al.* (1961) proposed tyrosines and carboxyls as ligands. Windle *et al.* (1963) and Aasa *et al.* (1963) both proposed histidines as essential groups, based on electron paramagnetic resonance studies showing nitrogen involvements. The nitrogen was shown not to be the amino nitrogen by chemical modification experiments (Buttkus *et al.*, 1965). Although tryptophans have been suggested as ligands (Tan and Woodworth, 1968, 1970), chemical modifications by Ford-

Hutchinson and Perkins (1972) did not indicate tryptophans to be involved. Tyrosines have been strongly implicated by several different chemical modifications (Komatsu and Feeney, 1967). Although the precise nature and number of ligands are not known, Windle et al. (1963) proposed a model for the iron complex in which 2 nitrogens from 2 histidines, 3 oxygens from 3 tyrosines, and a bicarbonate formed an octahedral complex with iron in the center.

Apparently the metal-binding of ovotransferrin does not result in a gross change in the structure of the protein, but rather in changes in more localized areas of the binding sites (Feeney and Allison, 1969; Tan, 1971). The colored iron complex, however, is more stable to heat and pressure, and more resistant to proteolytic enzymes and denaturing agents, than is the metal-free protein (Azari and Feeney, 1961; Tan and Woodworth, 1970).

Woodworth (1967) and Woodworth et al. (1969) supported the nonexistence of a 1 iron atom per 1 mole of ovotransferrin complex, but proposed the presence of a dimer of one molecule of iron-free ovotransferrin combined with one which has 2 iron per molecule. Aisen et al. (1970) and Williams et al. (1970), however, could not find evidence for a dimer. They proposed existence of ovotransferrin in three equilibrium forms: (1) iron free, (2) complex with 1 Fe^{3+}, and (3) complex with 2 Fe^{3+}.

The 2 atoms of Fe^{3+} are bound by 2 independent and equivalent specific sites on ovotransferrin (Aisen et al., 1966). The presence of 2 independent metal-binding sites, and the relatively large size of the protein (see Table I), have led to the idea of a possible subunit structure for ovotransferrin. However, Bezkorovainy et al. (1968) and Greene and Feeney (1968) concluded that ovotransferrin was a single polypeptide chain, based on their ultracentrifugation studies of samples in which the disulfides were reduced and the resulting sulfhydryls carboxymethylated. Greene and Feeney (1968) suggested that 2 homologous sections of a single chain originated by gene duplication and some type of fusion. Similar conclusions were reached by Phillips and Azari (1971) in their investigation of the products produced by cyanogen bromide cleavage of the methionyl residues. But Elleman and Williams (1970) identified more unique cysteic acid residues after performic acid oxidation than would be expected, based on identity of two similar sections. Their findings, however, do not preclude the existence of homology. Each original hypothetical half molecule could have undergone further mutational changes, or the original gene fusion might have been unequal. Frelinger (1972) has recently reported genetic studies with pigeons. He suggested that his results with the ovotransferrins indicated the existence of dimeric proteins, so that "hybrid" molecules could be produced in the heterozygote. But he also stated that differences in carbohydrate content could account for the observed differences.

As is generally the case with the other egg-white proteins, the biological function of ovotransferrin remains unknown. Although it is a potent inhibitor of microbial growth, as yet no evidence has been presented for any inhibitory effects in the higher animals.

VII. Ovoflavoprotein

A. History

The amount of riboflavin in the egg white was early shown to be directly influenced by the amount of riboflavin in the diet (Heiman, 1935; Norris and Bauernfeind, 1940). It was not until the report by Rhodes et al. (1958, 1959) that riboflavin was known to exist as a complex with a protein (apoprotein) to form the ovoflavoprotein in egg white. Rhodes and associates found that the capacity of riboflavin binding was not influenced by the amount of riboflavin in the hen's diet. Farrell et al. (1969) have more recently further characterized the ovoflavoprotein.

The absence of ovoflavoprotein in the eggs from a pedigreed flock of Single-Comb White Leghorn hens was due to an autosomal recessive gene (Maw, 1954). This lethal, hereditary malfunction could be corrected by the injection of riboflavin into the egg. Apparently the gene density directly dictated the amount of ovoflavoprotein in the egg white. A normal (RdRd) egg contained twice as much ovoflavoprotein as did the heterozygote (Rdrd); the one with the recessive allele (rdrd) contained little or no ovoflavoprotein

(Winter *et al.*, 1967). Farrell *et al.* (1970a) isolated and characterized the ovoflavoprotein from the egg whites produced by hens with the *RdRd* and *Rdrd* genotype. The chemical and physical properties of the ovoflavoprotein from the homozygote were essentially identical to those from the heterozygote. These investigators also showed that the flavoproteins from the serum, yolk, and white were seriologically identical (Farrell *et al.*, 1970b). However, although seriologically similar, the flavoprotein isolated and characterized from egg yolk by Ostrowski *et al.* (1968) had somewhat different chemical and physical properties from those of the flavoprotein from the egg white.

Clagett (1971) has recently reviewed certain aspects of his work on the White Leghorn hens, and has proposed a genetic control mechanism for the ovoflavoprotein.

B. General Physical, Chemical, and Biochemical Properties

The physical properties and chemical composition of ovoflavoprotein are listed in Tables I and II, respectively.

Rhodes *et al.* (1959) demonstrated that 1 mole of riboflavin was bound to 1 mole of apoprotein, and that no free flavin existed in the egg white. Unlike most flavoproteins, ovoflavoprotein did not contain either FMN or FAD. Binding experiments revealed that riboflavin was bound more tightly than FMN, FAD, and their analogs. Winter *et al.* (1967) and Becvar (1973) also reported that riboflavin was bound tightly ($K_{diss} = 10^{-6} M$ and $1.3 \times 10^{-9} M$). A yolk apoprotein appears to bind the flavin tightly ($K_{diss} = 2.65 \times 10^{-9} M$) (Ostrowski and Krawczyk, 1963).

Two ionic binding sites, and a possible subunit structure, have been implicated to be present in ovoflavoprotein (Farrell *et al.*, 1968). Farrell *et al.* (1969) reported that the binding site did not involve tyrosines or histidines, but that the tryptophan and carboxyl groups might be involved. Guanidine-HCl at 5 M concentration did affect the binding and this effect was reversible; the $s_{20,w}$ change from 3.0 to 1.7. Cotner and Clagett (1972) have isolated a fully active 24,000 gm subunit which may possibly contain a glycine at the COOH-terminal (Phillips *et al.*, 1969). Absorption spectra studies by Nishikimi and Yagi (1969) indicated that the flavin nucleus was buried in the hydrophobic region of the apoprotein. They also concluded by circular dichroism spectra that the riboflavin-apoprotein was fixed in a constant configuration from pH 4.5 to 9.0. The apoprotein did not lose any binding capacity after heating at 100°C for 15 minutes at pH 7, nor after 95% dephosphorylation by potato acid phosphatase (Rhodes *et al.*, 1959).

Rhodes *et al.* (1959) tested the antibacterial effect of apoprotein on *Streptococcus pyogenes* and *Lactobacillus casei*. Ten times the molar excess of apoprotein to riboflavin was necessary to cause complete inhibition of growth.

Bleumink and Young (1971) prepared samples of ovoflavoprotein–apoprotein by a method similar to that of Rhodes *et al.* (1959) and obtained a slight skin reaction from patients with egg-hypersensitivity. But the skin reaction was <3% of the skin reaction caused by purified ovomucoid.

Although at first appearance this riboflavin-binding protein might seem to be analogous to the biotin-binding protein avidin, this analogy might apply only to their similar functions of binding B vitamins and not to their nutritional effects. There is a very large difference ($>10^6$) in the strength of bindings, and no nutritional inhibitory effects have been observed with the riboflavin-binding protein, as in contrast to avidin.

Acknowledgment

The authors gratefully acknowledge advice and assistance from many individuals who supplied information used in this article.

References

Aasa, R., Malmstrom, B.G., Saltman, P., and Vanngard, T. (1963). *Biochim. Biophys. Acta* **75**, 203.

Abraham, E.P., and Robinson, R. (1937). *Nature (London)* **140**, 24.

Aisen, P., Leibman, A., and Reich, H.A. (1966). *J. Biol. Chem.* **241**, 1666.

Aisen, P., Aasa, R., Malmstrom, B.G., and Vanngard, T. (1967). *J. Biol. Chem.* **242**, 2484.

Aisen, P., Koenig, S.H., Schillinger, W.E., Scheinberg, I.H., Mann, K.G., and Fisk, W. (1970). *Nature (London)* **226**, 859.

Alderton, G., and Fevold, H.L. (1946). *J. Biol. Chem.* **164**, 1.

Alderton, G., Ward, W.H., and Fevold, H.L. (1946). *Arch. Biochem. Biophys.* **11**, 9.

Ankier, S.I. (1969). *Prog. Drug Res.* **13**, 341–394.

Arnheim, N., and Steller, R. (1970). *Arch. Biochem. Biophys.* **141**, 656.

Arnheim, N., and Wilson, A.C. (1967). *J. Biol. Chem.* **242**, 3451.

Arnheim, N., Prager, E.M., and Wilson, A.C. (1969). *J. Biol. Chem.* **244**, 2085.

Azari, P.R., and Feeney, R.E. (1961). *Arch. Biochem. Biophys.* **92**, 44.

Bain, J.A., and Deutsch, H.F. (1948). *J. Biol. Chem.* **172**, 547.

Baker, C.M.A. (1968). *In* "Egg Quality, A Study of Hen's Eggs" (T.C. Carter, ed.), No. 4, pp. 67–108. Oliver & Boyd, Edinburgh.

Baker, C.M.A. (1970), *Advan. Genet.* **15**, 147.

Baker, C.M.A., and Manwell, C. (1967). *Comp. Biochem. Physiol.* **23**, 21.

Ball, H.R., and Cotterill, O.J. (1971a). *Poultry Sci.* **50**, 435.

Ball, H.R., and Cotterill, O.J. (1971b). *Poultry Sci.* **50**, 446.

Becvar, J.E. (1973). Ph.D. Thesis. Univ. of Michigan.

Beeley, J.G. (1971). *Biochem. J.* **123**, 399.

Beeley, J.G., and Jevons, F.R. (1965). *Biochim. Biophys. Acta* **101**, 133.

Bezkorovainy, A., Grohlich, D., and Gerbeck, C.M. (1968). *Biochem. J.* **110**, 765.

Blake, C.C.F., Koening, D.F., Mair, G.A., North, A.C.T., Phillips, D.C., and Sarma, V.R. (1965). *Nature (London)* **206**, 757.

Blake, C.C.F., Johnson, L.N., Mair, G.A., North, A.C.T., Phillips, D.C., and Sarma, V.R. (1967). *Proc. Roy. Soc., Ser. B* **167**, 378.

Bleumink, E., and Young, E. (1969). *Int. Arch. Allergy Appl. Immunol.* **35**, 1.

Bleumink, E., and Young, E. (1971). *Int. Arch. Allergy Appl. Immunol.* **40**, 72.

Boas, M.A. (1924). *Biochem. J.* **18**, 422.

Boas, M.A. (1927). *Biochem. J.* **21**, 712.

Boyd, E.M., and Sargeant, E.J. (1962). *J. New Drugs* **2**, 283.

Buck, F.F., Bier, M., and Nord, F.F. (1962). *Arch. Biochem. Biophys.* **98**, 528.

Buttkus, H., Clark, J.R., and Feeney, R.E. (1965). *Biochemistry* **6**, 1136.

Canfield, R.E. (1963). *J. Biol. Chem.* **238**, 2698.

Canfield, R.E., and Anfinsen, C.G. (1963). *Biochemistry* **2**, 1073.

Canfield, R.E., Kammerman, S., Sabel, J.H., and Morgan, F.J. (1971). *Nature (London) New Biol.* **232**, 16.

Chipman, D.M., and Sharon, N. (1969). *Science* **165**, 454.

Clagett, C.O. (1971). *Fed. Proc., Fed. Amer. Soc. Exp. Biol.* **30**, 127.

Cotner, R.C., and Clagett, C.O. (1972). *Fed. Proc., Fed. Amer. Soc. Exp. Biol.* **31**, 851.

Cuatrecasas, P., and Wilchek, M. (1968). *Biochem. Biophys. Res. Commun.* **33**, 235.

Cunha, T.J., Lindley, D.C., and Ensminger, M.E. (1946). *J. Anim. Sci.* **5**, 219.

Davis, J.G., Zahnley, J.C., and Donovan, J.W. (1969). *Biochemistry* **8**, 2044.

DeLange, R.J. (1970). *J. Biol. Chem.* **245**, 907.

DeLange, R.J., and Huang, T.S. (1971). *J. Biol. Chem.* **246**, 698.

Delezene, C., and Pozerski, E. (1904). *C. R. Soc. Biol.* **55**, 935.

Donovan, J.W., and Hansen, L.U. (1971a). *J. Food Sci.* **36**, 174.

Donovan, J.W., and Hansen, L.U. (1971b). *J. Food Sci.* **36,** 178.
Donovan, J.W., and Ross, K.D. (1972). *Fed. Proc., Fed. Amer. Soc. Exp. Biol.* **31,** 469.
Donovan, J.W., Mapes, C.J., Davis, J.G., and Hamburg, R.D. (1969). *Biochemistry* **8,** 4190.
Donovan, J.W., Davis, J.G., and White, L.M. (1970). *Biochim. Biophys. Acta* **207,** 190.
Eakin, R.E., Snell, E.E., and Williams, R.J. (1940a). *J. Biol. Chem.* **136,** 801.
Eakin, R.E., Snell, E.E., and Williams, R.J. (1940b). *Science* **92,** 224.
Eakin, R.E., Snell, E.E., and Williams, R.J. (1941). *J. Biol. Chem.* **140,** 535.
Elleman, T.C., and Williams, J. (1970). *Biochem. J.* **116,** 515.
Farrell, H.M., Mallette, M.F., and Clagett, C.O. (1968). *Fed. Proc., Fed. Amer. Soc. Exp. Biol.* **27,** 456.
Farrell, H.M., Mallette, M.F., Buss, E.G., and Clagett, C.O. (1969). *Biochim. Biophys. Acta* **194,** 433.
Farrell, H.M., Buss, E.G., and Clagett, C.O. (1970a). *Int. J. Biochem.* **1,** 157.
Farrell, H.M., Buss, E.G., and Clagett, C.O. (1970b). *Int. J. Biochem.* **1,** 168.
Faure, A., and Jolles, P. (1970). *FEBS Lett.* **10,** 237.
Feeney, R.E. (1971a). *In* "Proceedings of the International Research Conference on Proteinase Inhibitors" (H. Fritz and H. Tschesche, eds.), pp. 162–168. deGruyter, Berlin.
Feeney, R.E. (1971b). *In* "Proceedings of the International Research Conference on Proteinase Inhibitors" (H. Fritz and H. Tschesche, eds.), pp. 189–195. de Gruyter, Berlin.
Feeney, R.E., and Allison, R.G. (1969). "Evolutionary Biochemistry of Proteins." Wiley (Interscience), New York.
Feeney, R.E., and Komatsu, S.K. (1966). *In* "Structure and Bonding" (C.K. Jergensen *et al.*, eds.), Vol. 1, pp. 149–206. Springer-Verlag, Berlin and New York.
Feeney, R.E., MacDonnell, L.R., and Ducay, E.D. (1956). *Arch. Biochem. Biophys.* **61,** 72.
Feeney, R.E., Stevens, F.C., and Osuga, D.T. (1963). *J. Biol. Chem.* **238,** 1415.
Feeney, R.E., Osuga, D.T., and Maeda, H. (1967). *Arch. Biochem. Biophys.* **119,** 124.
Feeney, R.E., Allison, R.G., Osuga, D.T., Bigler, J.C., and Miller, H.T. (1968). *In* "Antarctic Research Series" (O.L. Austin, ed.), Vol. 12, pp. 151–165. Amer. Geophys. Union, Washington, D.C.
Feeney, R.E., Means, G.E., and Bigler, J.C. (1969). *J. Biol. Chem.* **244,** 1957.
Feeney, R.E., Rhodes, M.B., and Anderson, J.S. (1960). *J. Biol. Chem.* **235,** 2633.
Feinstein, G., and Feeney, R.E. (1966). *J. Biol. Chem.* **241,** 5183.
Fernandez Diaz, M.J., Osuga, D.T., and Feeney, R.E. (1964). *Arch. Biochem. Biophys.* **107,** 449.
Fevold, H.L. (1951). *Advan. Protein Chem.* **6,** 187.
Fleming, A. (1922). *Proc. Roy. Soc. Ser. B* **93,** 306.
Ford-Hutchinson, A.W., and Perkins, D.J. (1972). *Eur. J. Biochem.* **25,** 415.
Fossum, K., and Whitaker, J.R. (1968). *Arch. Biochem. Biophys.* **125,** 367.
Fraenkel-Conrat, H., and Feeney, R.E. (1950). *Arch. Biochem.* **29,** 101.
Fraenkel-Conrat, H., and Porter, R.R. (1952). *Biochim. Biophys. Acta* **9,** 557.

Fraenkel-Conrat, H., Snell, N.S., and Ducay, E.D. (1952a). *Arch. Biochem. Biophys.* **39**, 80.
Fraenkel-Conrat, H., Snell, N.S., and Ducay, E.D. (1952b). *Arch. Biochem. Biophys.* **39**, 97.
Frelinger, J.A. (1972). *Proc. Nat. Acad. Sci. U.S.* **69**, 326.
Gertler, A., and Feinstein, G. (1971). *Eur. J. Biochem.* **20**, 547.
Gottschalk, A., and Lind, P.E. (1959). *Brit. J. Exp. Pathol.* **30**, 85.
Green, N.M. (1962). *Biochim. Biophys. Acta.* **59**, 244.
Green, N.M. (1963a). *Biochem. J.* **89**, 585.
Green, N.M. (1963b). *Biochem. J.* **89**, 591.
Green, N.M. (1963c). *Biochem. J.* **89**, 599.
Green, N.M. (1963d). *Biochem. J.* **89**, 609.
Green, N.M. (1964a). *Biochem. J.* **90**, 564.
Green, N.M. (1964b). *Biochem. J.* **92**, 16c.
Green, N.M. (1965). *Biochem. J.* **94**, 23c.
Green, N.M. (1966). *Biochem. J.* **101**, 774.
Green, N.M. (1967). *Biochem. J.* **104**, 64p.
Green, N.M. (1968). *Nature (London)* **217**, 254.
Green, N.M. (1970a). *In* "Methods in Enzymology" (D.B. McCormick and L.D. Wright, eds.), Vol. 18, Part A, pp. 414–417. Academic Press, New York.
Green, N.M. (1970b). *In* "Methods in Enzymology" (D.B. McCormick and L.D. Wright, eds.), Vol. 18, Part A, pp. 418–424. Academic Press, New York.
Green, N.M., and Joynson, M.A. (1970). *Biochem. J.* **118**, 71.
Green, N.M., and Melamed, M.D. (1966). *Biochem. J.* **100**, 614.
Green, N.M., and Ross, M.E. (1968). *Biochem. J.* **110**, 59.
Green, N.M., and Toms, E.J. (1970). *Biochem. J.* **118**, 67.
Green, N.M., Konieczny, L., Toms, E.J., and Valentine, R.C. (1971). *Biochem. J.* **125**, 781.
Greene, F.C., and Feeney, R.E. (1968). *Biochemistry* **7**, 1366.
György, P. (1954). *In* "The Vitamins" (W.H. Sebrell, Jr. and R.S. Harris, eds.), 1st ed., Vol. 1, pp. 600–613. Academic Press, New York.
György, P., and Rose, C.S. (1941). *Science* **94**, 261.
György, P., and Rose, C.S. (1943). *Proc. Soc. Exp. Biol. Med.* **53**, 55.
Haynes, R., Osuga, D.T., and Feeney, R.E. (1967). *Biochemistry* **6**, 541.
Hedin, S.G. (1907). *Hoppe-Seyler's Z. Physiol. Chem.* **52**, 412.
Heiman, V. (1935). *Poultry Sci.* **14**, 137.
Hermann, J., and Jollès, J. (1970). *Biochim. Biophys. Acta* **200**, 178.
Hermann, J., Jollès, J., and Jollès, P. (1971). *Eur. J. Biochem.* **24**, 12.
Huang, T.S., and DeLange, R.J. (1971). *J. Biol. Chem.* **246**, 686.
Isemura, T., Takagi, T., Maeda, Y., and Imai, K. (1961). *Biochem. Biophys. Res. Commun.* **5**, 373.
Jollès, J., Jaurequi-Adell, J., Bernier, I., and Jollès, P. (1963). *Biochim. Biophys. Acta* **78**, 668.
Jollès, J., Spotorno, G., and Jollès, P. (1965). *Nature (London)* **208**, 1204.
Jollès, J., van Leemputten, E., Mouton, A., and Jollès, P. (1972). *Biochim. Biophys. Acta* **257**, 497.

Jollès, P. (1964). *Angew Chem. Int. Ed. Engl.* **3**, 28.

Kaneda, M., Kato, I., Tominaga, N., Titani, K., and Narita, K. (1969). *J. Biochim. (Tokyo)* **66**, 747.

Kassell, B. (1970). *In* "Methods in Enzymology" (G.E. Perlmann and L. Lorand, eds.), Vol. 19, pp. 839–906. Academic Press, New York.

Ketterer, B. (1962). *Life Sci.* **5**, 163.

Ketterer, B. (1965). *Biochem. J.* **96**, 372.

Klose, A.A., Hill, B., and Fevold, H.L. (1950). *Arch. Biochem.* **27**, 364.

Komatsu, S.K., and Feeney, R.E. (1967). *Biochemistry* **6**, 1136.

Korenman, S.G., and O'Malley, B.W. (1967). *Biochim. Biophys. Acta* **140**, 174.

Korenman, S.G., and O'Malley, B.W. (1970). *In* "Methods in Enzymology" (D.B. McCormick and L.D. Wright, eds.), Vol. 18, Part A, pp. 427–430. Academic Press, New York.

La Rue, J.N., and Speck, J.C., Jr. (1970). *J. Biol. Chem.* **245**, 1985.

Laschtschenko, P. (1909). *Z. Hyg. Infektionskr.* **64**, 419.

Laskowski, M., and Laskowski, M., Jr. (1954). *Advan. Protein Chem.* **9**, 203.

Laskowski, M., Jr., Duran, R.W., Finkenstadt, W.R., Herbert, S., Hixson, H.F., Jr., Kowalski, D., Luthy, J.A., Mattis, J.A., McKee, R.E., and Niekamp, C.W. (1971). *In* "Proceedings of the International Research Conference on Proteinase Inhibitors" (H. Fritz and H. Tschesche, eds.), pp. 117–134. de Gruyter, Berlin.

Liener, I.E., and Kakade, M.L. (1969). *In* "Toxic Constituents of Plant Foodstuffs" (I. E. Liener, ed.), pp. 7–68. Academic Press, New York.

Light, R.A. (1951). *Surgery* **30**, 195.

Lin, Y., and Feeney, R.E. (1972). *In* "Glycoproteins" (A. Gottschalk, ed.), 2nd ed., pp. 762–781. Elsevier, Amsterdam.

Linderstrom-Lang, K., and Ottesen, M. (1947). *Nature (London)* **159**, 807.

Lineweaver, H., and Murray, C.W. (1947). *J. Biol. Chem.* **171**, 565.

Liu, W. H., Feinstein, G., Osuga, D. T., Haynes, R., and Feeney, R. E. (1968). *Biochemistry* **7**, 2886.

Liu, W. H., Means, G. E., and Feeney, R. E. (1971). *Biochim. Biophys. Acta* **229**, 176.

Lobstein, O.E. (1961). *Symp. Int. Lisozima Fleming, 2nd, 1961.*

Longsworth, L.G., Cannon, R.K., and MacInnes, D.A. (1940). *J. Amer. Chem. Soc.* **62**, 2580.

McCormick, D. B. (1965). *Anal. Biochem.* **13**, 194.

MacDonnell, L. R., Silva, R. B., and Feeney, R. E. (1951). *Arch. Biochem. Biophys.* **32**, 288.

Matsushima, K. (1958a). *J. Agr. Chem. Soc. Jap.* **32**, 211.

Matsushima, K. (1958b). *Science* **127**, 1178.

Maw, A.J.G. (1954). *Poultry Sci.* **33**, 216.

Melamed, M.D. (1966). *In* "Glycoproteins" (A. Gottschalk, ed.), pp. 317–334. Amer. Elsevier, New York.

Melamed, M. D., and Green, N. M. (1963). *Biochem. J.* **89**, 591.

Meyer, K. (1945). *Advan. Protein Chem.* **2**, 264.

Miller, H., and Campbell, D.H. (1950). *J. Allergy* **21**, 522.

Miller, H. T., and Feeney, R. E. (1964). *Arch. Biochem. Biophys.* **108**, 117.

Miller, H. T., and Feeney, R. E. (1966). *Biochemistry* **5**, 952.

Morner, C. T. (1894). *Hoppe-Seylers Z. Physiol. Chem.* **18,** 525.
Nishikimi, M., and Yagi, K. (1969). *J. Biochem. (Tokyo)* **66,** 427.
Norris, L. C., and Bauernfeind, J. C. (1940). *Food Res.* **5,** 521.
O'Malley, B. W., and Korenman, S. G. (1967). *Life Sci.* **6,** 1953.
Osborne, T. B., and Campbell, G. F. (1900). *J. Amer. Chem. Soc.* **22,** 422.
Ostrowski, W., and Krawczyk, A. (1963). *Acta Chem. Scand.* **17,** S241.
Ostrowski, W., Zak, Z., and Krawczyk, A. (1968). *Acta Biochim. Pol.* **15,** 242.
Osuga, D. T., and Feeney, R. E. (1968). *Biochim. Biophys. Acta* **159,** 209.
Ottesen, M. (1958). *C. R. Trav. Lab. Carlsberg* **30,** 211.
Ozawa, K., and Laskowski, M., Jr. (1966). *J. Biol. Chem.* **241,** 3955.
Pai, C. H., and Lichstein, H. C. (1964). *Proc. Soc. Exp. Biol. Med.* **116,** 197.
Parsons, H. T., and Kelly, E. (1933a). *Amer. J. Physiol.* **104,** 150.
Parsons, H. T., and Kelly, E. (1933b). *J. Biol. Chem.* **100,** 645.
Parsons, H.T., Gardner, J., and Walliker, C.T. (1940). *J. Nut.* **19,** Suppl., 19 *(abstr.)*
Pearlman, G. E. (1952). *J. Gen. Physiol.* **25,** 711.
Pennington, D., Snell, E. E., and Eakin, R. E. (1942). *J. Amer. Chem. Soc.* **64,** 469.
Peters, J. M. (1967). *Brit. J. Nutr.* **21,** 801.
Peters, J. M., and Boyd, E. M. (1966). *Toxicol. Appl. Pharmacol.* **8,** 350.
Phillips, D. C. (1967). *Proc. Int. Cong. Biochem.* **36,** 63.
Phillips, J. L., and Azari, P. (1971). *Biochemistry* **10,** 1160.
Phillips, J.W., Mallette, M.F., and Clagett, C.O. (1969). *Fed. Proc., Fed. Amer. Soc. Exp. Biol.* **28,** 888.
Prager, E. M., and Wilson, A. C. (1971a). *J. Biol. Chem.* **246,** 523.
Prager, E. M., and Wilson, A. C. (1971b). *J. Biol. Chem.* **246,** 5978.
Prager, E. M., and Wilson, A. C. (1971c). *J. Biol. Chem.* **246,** 7010.
Price, E.M., and Gibson, J.F. (1972). *Biochem. Biophys. Res. Commun.* **46,** 646.
Pritchard, A.B., McCormick, D.B., and Wright, L.D. (1966). *Biochem. Biophys. Res. Commun.* **25,** 524.
Raftery, M. A., and Dahlquist, F. W. (1969). *Fortschr. Chem. Org. Naturst.* **27,** 340.
Rauch, H., and Nutting, W. B. (1958). *Experientia* **14,** 382.
Rhodes, M. B., Azari, P. R., and Feeney, R. E. (1958). *J. Biol. Chem.* **230,** 399.
Rhodes, M. B., Bennett, N., and Feeney, R. E. (1959). *J. Biol. Chem.* **234,** 2054.
Rhodes, M. B., Adams, J. L., Bennett, N., and Feeney, R. E. (1960a). *Poultry Sci.* **39,** 1473.
Rhodes, M. B., Bennett, N., and Feeney, R. E. (1960b). *J. Biol. Chem.* **235,** 1686.
Robinson, D. S., and Monsey, J. B. (1971). *Biochem. J.* **121,** 537.
Salton, M. R. J. (1964). "The Bacteria Cell Wall." Elsevier, Amsterdam.
Schade, A. L., and Caroline, L. (1944). *Science* **100,** 14.
Schade, A. L., Reinhart, R. W., and Levy, H. (1949). *Arch. Biochem.* **20,** 170.
Scudamore, H. H., Morey, G. R., Consolozio, C. F., Berryman, G. H., Gordon, L. E., Lightbody, H. D., and Fevold, H. L. (1949). *J. Nutr.* **39,** 555.
Smith, M. B. (1964). *Aust. J. Biol. Sci.* **17,** 261.
Snell, E. E., Eakin, R. E., and Williams, R. J. (1940). *J. Amer. Chem. Soc.* **62,** 175.
Sophianapoulos, A. J., and Van Holde, K. E. (1964). *J. Biol. Chem.* **239,** 2516.
Spande, T. F., Witkop, B., Degani, Y., and Patchornik, A. (1970). *Advan. Protein Chem.* **24,** 98.

Stevens, F. C., and Feeney, R. E. (1963). *Biochemistry* **2**, 1346.

Sri, Ram, Terminiello, J. L., Bier, M., and Nord, F. F. (1954). *Arch. Biochem. Biophys.* **52**, 451.

Sydenstricker, V. P., Singal, S. A., Briggs, A. P., DeVaughn, N. M., and Isabell, H. (1942). *Science* **95**, 176.

Tan, A. T. (1971). *Can. J. Biochem.* **49**, 1071.

Tan, A. T., and Woodworth, R. C. (1968). *Fed. Proc., Fed. Amer. Soc. Exp. Biol.* **27**, 780.

Tan, A. T., and Woodworth, R. C. (1969). *Biochemistry* **8**, 3711.

Tan, A. T., and Woodworth, R. C. (1970). *J. Polym. Sci. 30C*, 599.

Thompson, R. (1940). *Arch. Pathol.* **30**, 1096.

Tomimatsu, Y., Clary, J. J., and Bartulovich, J. J. (1966). *Arch. Biochem. Biophys.* **115**, 536.

Vaughan, J. H. and Kabat, E. A. (1954). *J. Allergy* **25**, 387.

Vogel, R., Trautschold, I., and Werle, E. (1969). "Natural Proteinase Inhibitors." Academic Press, New York.

Warner, R. C. (1954). *In* "The Proteins" (H. Neurath and K. Bailey, eds.), 1st ed., Vol. 2, Part A, pp. 435–485. Academic Press, New York.

Warner, R. C., and Weber, I. (1951). *J. Biol. Chem.* **191**, 173.

Warner, R. C., and Weber, I. (1953). *J. Amer. Chem. Soc.* **75**, 5094.

Wei, R. D. (1970). *In* "Methods in Enzymology" (D. B. McCormick and L. D. Wright, eds.), Vol. 18, Part A, pp. 424–427. Academic Press, New York.

Wei, R. D., and Wright, L. D. (1964). *Proc. Soc. Exp. Biol. Med.* **117**, 17.

Williams, J. (1962). *Biochem. J.* **83**, 355.

Williams, J., Phelps, C. F., and Lowe, J. M. (1970). *Nature (London)* **226**, 858.

Windle, J. J., Wiersema, A. K., Clark, J. R., and Feeney, R. E. (1963). *Biochemistry* **2**, 1341.

Winter, W. P., Buss, E. G., Clagett, C. O., and Boucher, R. V. (1967). *Comp. Biochem. Physiol.* **22**, 897.

Wishnia, A., Weber, I., and Warner, R. C. (1961). *J. Amer. Chem. Soc.* **83**, 2071.

Woodworth, R.C. (1967). *Peptides Biol. Fluids* **14**, 37.

Woodworth, R. C., Tan, A. T., and Virkaitis, L. R. (1969). *Nature (London)* **223**, 833.

Woolley, D. W., and Longsworth, L. G. (1942). *J. Biol. Chem.* **142**, 285.

Wright, L. D. Valentik, K. A., Nepple, M. H. Cresson, E. L., and Skeggs, H. R. (1950). *Proc. Soc. Exp. Biol. Med.* **74**, 273.

3

□ □ □

FISH EGGS

Frederick A. Fuhrman

I. Introduction

It has been known for several thousand years that the eggs of
certain fish are poisonous when eaten. The earliest Chinese
pharmacopeia, *Pen-T'so Chin* or *The Herbal,* which dates from the
first or second century B.C. or earlier, included the eggs of puffer
fish among its drugs (cf. Kao, 1966). The first experimental confirmation that eggs of certain fish are poisonous was recorded in a
book entitled "Corona Florida Medicinae" by Antonio Gazio and
published in Venice in 1491. He states that according to popular
opinion the eggs of the barbel (probably *Barbus meridionalis)* should
not be eaten. To test the validity of this folk knowledge he ate some
and several hours later suffered vomiting and diarrhea (cf. Halstead, 1965). Although almost five hundred years have passed
since Gazio's experiment, most of the toxins from fish eggs, with
the notable exception of tetrodotoxin, are still poorly characterized
and the nature of the intoxications is obscure. These toxins have
been termed *ichthyoötoxins* to distinguish them from other toxins
that are distributed throughout the tissues of fish (cf. Halstead,
1967). The reason for the occurrence of toxins in the eggs of fish is
conjectural. It seems reasonable that it should discourage predators and therefore be of value to the survival of the species. It certainly has served to discourage gourmets from indulging in some
kinds of caviar.

A. TYPES OF POISONING FROM FISH EGGS

Poisoning caused by eating fish eggs containing naturally occurring toxins may be divided into three general types. By far the
most important of these is tetrodotoxin poisoning caused by eating
the roe of puffer fish, or *fugu,* which contain tetrodotoxin.The
symptoms of poisoning occur within a few minutes, progress rapidly from tingling and numbness of the tongue and lips to muscular
paralysis, and, in about 50% of the cases, to death from respiratory
paralysis. A completely different form of poisoning occurs after
eating the roe of two species of marine fish, the northern blenny
(Stichaeus grigorgjewi) and the cabezon *(Scorpaenichthys marmoratus).*

The symptoms appear after 6–12 hours, and include vomiting, diarrhea, headache, chest pain, dizziness, and occasionally coma and death. The toxins are lipoproteins. A third type of poisoning occurs after eating the eggs of a number of freshwater fishes such as the barbel, pike, and gar. Symptoms appear earlier than after lipoprotein poisoning, and are much less severe, consisting of nausea, vomiting, and diarrhea. The nature of the toxins involved is obscure.

B. Fish-borne Botulism and Other Forms of Food Poisoning from Fish Eggs

Certain types of bacterial food poisoning usually result in nausea, vomiting, diarrhea, and prostration and hence may be mistaken for poisoning produced by ingestion of fish eggs containing a naturally occurring toxin of type 2 or 3 in the classification given above. Such food poisoning may result either from toxins produced by bacteria that have grown on foods such as fish eggs (e.g., staphylococci), or from infection with the bacteria themselves that multiply in the human intestine (e.g., salmonella and *Clostridium welchii*) (cf. Taylor and McCoy, 1969).

Fish-borne botulism is of particular interest because several outbreaks have been caused by eating fish eggs, and because the epidemiology is quite clear. Both botulism and tetrodon poisoning produce paralysis and may perhaps be confused, although the onset of the former is much slower. The older European medical literature contains many reports of a special kind of poisoning designated paralytic ichthyism or *Fischvergiftung* that followed eating various fish products, including fish eggs, and that clearly differed in symptomology from that caused by the usual bacteria (cf. Rieman, 1969). A particularly lucid account was given by Schreiber (1884) of such poisoning of six members of a single family, two of whom died several days after eating preserved fish. The symptoms included weakness, headache, difficulty in swallowing, diplopia, muscular paralysis, and respiratory failure. Clearly, this outbreak as well as others in the literature (cf. Witthaus, 1911) were fish-borne botulism, as gradually became apparent to

Russian pathologists around 1900 (Zlatogoroff and Soloviev, 1927; Dolman and Chang, 1953). Botulism attributable to fish eggs is usually caused by the type E strain of *Clostridium botulinum*, a designation first applied to cultures isolated from the intestines and muscle of sturgeon from the Sea of Azov (Gunnison *et al.*, 1936). It has now been demonstrated that type E *CL. botulinum* can be cultured from the intestinal contents of many fish, and from the mud of rivers and sand of harbors and of the sea in many parts of the northern hemisphere (cf. Dolman, 1957; Herzberg, 1970). For example, in the mud from Copenhagen harbor the incidence was 17% in 34 samples (Pedersen, 1955), while in that from Green Bay of Lake Michigan it was 97% in 64 samples (Sugiyama *et al.*, 1970). Dolman *et al.* (1960) have described in detail two outbreaks of botulism (one type E and one type B) in British Columbia caused by eating salmon eggs. Sakaguchi (1969) summarized 10 outbreaks of botulism caused by fish eggs. The mortality rate was about 50%. The presence of spores in the soil, water, and fish constitute a hazard to inhabitants of those countries such as Alaska, Japan, Russia, and Western Canada where uncooked fish eggs are commonly eaten. It is a tribute to the efficiency of the methods used by the Russian caviar industry that for many years there have been no reports of botulism caused by these preserved sturgeon eggs.

II. Tetrodotoxin

A. HISTORY AND OCCURRENCE

It has been known for thousands of years that the ovaries, eggs and liver of various fishes belonging to the order Tetraodontiformes, commonly known as puffers, globefish, swellfish, or *fugu* (Fig. 1), are poisonous when eaten. Macht (1942) suggests that the prohibition against eating scaleless fish in the Mosaic sanitary laws was directed at puffers. Certainly the toxicity of puffer eggs has been known in the Orient for a very long time. As already mentioned, they were included among the 365 drugs in *Pen-T'so Chin* or *The Herbal* (ca. second century B. C.), where they were recommended to arrest convulsive diseases (cf. Kao, 1966). In a Chinese treatise by Chaun Yanfang written during the Sui Dynasty (A.D. 581–617), entitled "Studies on the Origins of Diseases," an accurate account is given of the toxicity of the liver, eggs, and ovaries of the puffer fish (Tani, 1945). Knowledge of these poisonous fish reached Europe early in the eighteenth century with the publication of Englebert Kaempfer's *History of Japan* (1727). Soon thereafter many accounts of the poisonous nature of the tetrodon fish were published by travelers to India, China, Japan, the Philippines, and Mexico. The monograph by Halstead (1967) and the review by Kao (1966) may be consulted for more detailed history of puffer poisoning.

The symptoms of tetrodon poisoning in man were accurately described by Captain James Cook in the journals of his second voyage around the world in the *Resolution* (Beagelhole, 1961). The ship's clerk obtained a fish from a native, and Cook asked that the fish be prepared for supper which he was to share with the expedition's two naturalists, J. R. Forster and Georg Forster. However, so much time was spent in drawing and describing the fish that only the roe and liver were cooked, and the three men ate sparingly. Cook wrote:

> About 3 or 4 o'clock in the Morning we were seized with an extraordinary weakness in all our limbs attended with a numbness or Sensation like to that caused by exposeing ones hands or feet to a fire after having been pinched by frost. I had almost lost the sence of feeling nor could I distinguish between light and heavy bodies, a quart pot full of Water and a feather was the same in my hand.

The naturalists identified the fish as belonging to the genus *Tetrodon,* and it is fortunate that Cook and his companions did in fact eat sparingly of it.

In the late nineteenth century attempts were made in Japan to isolate the toxic substance from the ovaries of various puffer fish. In 1910 Tahara announced the "purification" of an extract of these eggs which he named *tetrodotoxin,* and which had a lethal dose of about 7mg/kg. We now know that this product was about 0.15% pure, but it served as the material on which much of the early pharmacological studies were made. In 1950 Yokoo reported the

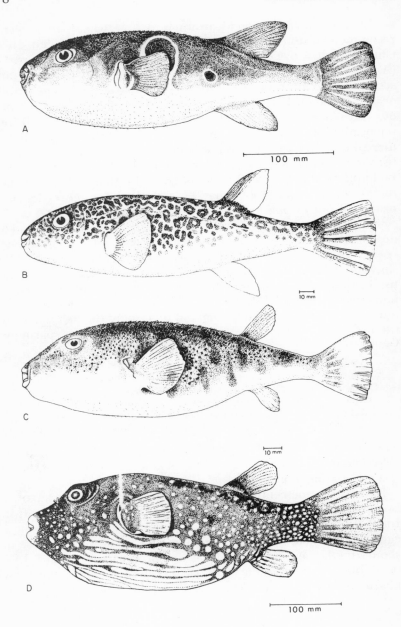

isolation of a crystalline toxin from the ovaries of *Sphaeroides* (=*Fugu*) *rubripes* which he named spheroidine. The name tetrodotoxin, however, is now universally used for the crystalline toxin.

Tetrodotoxin occurs in only one group of animals other than the tetrodon fishes. These are newts of the family Salamandridae (cf. Mosher *et al.,* 1964). This surprising finding came about as the result of grafting experiments on newts begun at Stanford University in the early 1930's by Professor Victor Twitty. He and his colleagues found that when eye vesicles of the local newt *Taricha* (formerly *Triturus*) *torosa* were transplanted into embryos of the tiger salamander *Ambystoma tigrinum,* the host became paralyzed. Twitty correctly concluded that the embryos of *Taricha* must contain a toxin capable of paralyzing *Ambystoma,* and soon a rather crude, but pharmacologically active, toxin was obtained from newt eggs (Van Wagtendonk *et al.,* 1942). Twenty years later this toxin was obtained in crystalline form (Brown and Mosher, 1963).As further studies were made of its chemical and pharmacological properties, it became clear that this toxin was identical with tetrodotoxin (Buchwald *et al.,* 1964). Thus, tetrodotoxin occurs in the eggs (and certain other organs) of fishes of the order Tetraodontiformes and newts of the family Salamandridae. No other animals are known to contain the toxin.*

B. FISHES CONTAINING TETRODOTOXIN

About 80 fishes of the order Tetraodontiformes are known to contain, or are suspected of containing tetrodotoxin. Lists of these are given by Kao (1966), Halstead (1967), and Bouder *et al.* (1962).

*Note added in proof: Noguchi and Hashimoto (1973) have now isolated crystalline tetrodotoxin from a fish not related to the puffers, a Goby, *Gobius criniger.*

Fig. 1. Puffer fish, or globefish, belonging to the order Tetraodontiformes. The eggs contain tetrodotoxin. (A) *Fugu rubripes rubripes* (Temminck and Schlegel). A common puffer known as *Torafugu* in Japan. It is highly prized for food. (B) *Fugu vermicularis vermicularis* (Temminck and Schlegel). A common puffer used for food in Japan. (C) *Sphaeroides maculatus* (Bloch and Schneider). The common puffer of the Atlantic coast of North America. (D) *Arothron hispidus* (Linnaeus). This puffer is widely distributed throughout the tropical seas. It has been responsible for poisoning in Hawaii, the Philippines and countries bordering the Red Sea.

TABLE I

Puffers and Related Fish Shown to Have Poisonous Eggs and Ovaries

Order: Tetraodontiformes

	Distribution[a]	Reference
Family: Canthigasteridae (Sharp-nosed puffers)		
Canthigaster rivulatus Timminck and Schlegel	A	Tani (1945); Takahashi and Inoko (1892)
Family: Diodontidae (Porcupine fish)		
Chilomycterus sp.	A	Halstead and Schall (1955)
Diodon hystrix Linnaeus	B	F. A. Fuhrman and G. J. Fuhrman (unpublished observations, 1966)
Family: Tetraodontidae (Puffers, swellfish, fugu)		
Arothron hispidus Linnaeus	B	Halstead and Schall (1955); Goe and Halstead (1953)
Arothron meleagris Lacepede	A	Halstead and Bunker (1954)
Arothron setosus Smith	C	Halstead and Schall (1956)
Fugu basilevskianus Basilewsky	D	Tani (1945)
Fugu chrysops Hilgendorf	D	Takahashi and Inoko (1892); Tani (1945)

Species	Distribution	References
Fugu niphobles Jordan and Snyder	D	Tani (1945)
Fugu ocellatus Linnaeus	D	Tani (1945)
Fugu paradalis Temminck and Schlegel	D	Tani (1945)
Fugu poecilonotus Temminck and Schlegel	A	Takahashi and Inoko (1892); Tani (1945)
Fugu pseudommus Chu	D	Tani (1945)
Fugu rubripes Temminck and Schlegel	D	Tani (1945)
Fugu stictonotus Temminck and Schlegel	D	Tani (1945)
Fugu vermicularis porphyreus Temminck and Schlegel	D	Takahashi and Inoko (1892); Tani (1945)
Fugu vermicularis radiatus Abe	D	Hashimoto (1950): Halstead and Bunker (1953)
Fugu vermicularis vermicularis Temminck and Schlegel	D	Takahashi and Inoko (1892); Halstead and Bunker (1953); Tani (1945)
Fugu xanthopterus Temminck and Schlegel	D	Tani (1945)
Lagocephalus sceleratus Forster	A	Tani (1945)
Sphaeroides annulatus Jenyns	C	Lalone et al. (1963); Halstead and Goe (1953); Halstead and Schall (1955)
Sphaeroides maculatus Bloch and Schneider	E	Larson et al. (1960); Yudkin (1945); Lalone et al. (1963)
Sphaeroides testudineus Linnaeus	E	Larson et al. (1960)

[a] Key to Distribution (based on Halstead, 1967, and Fish and Cobb, 1954): (A) Pacific and Indian Oceans; (B) worldwide tropical seas; (C) west coast of California and Mexico; (D) China Sea and Japan; (E) Atlantic coast of United States and eastward.

Those fish for which there is definite positive evidence of the presence of a toxin in the eggs or ovaries are listed in Table I. The classification and terminology is that of Halstead (1967). It should be noted that the genus *Fugu* is used for many of the Japanese puffers formerly classified in the genera *Tetrodon* and *Sphaeroides*.

It is of interest that fish belonging to three families of the order Tetraodontiformes have been found to have toxic eggs or ovaries. Only in a few species has it been shown that this toxin is, in fact, tetrodotoxin, but there is no evidence that any other toxin is present in these tissues, so we may assume that the toxicity is indeed due to tetrodotoxin. It is to be expected that fish belonging to these families other than those listed in Table I also have toxic eggs and ovaries, but this has not yet been established. In certain instances, however, it has been shown that the ovaries of some tetrodon fish are nontoxic. Tani (1945) used an assay method consisting of extraction, concentration, and injection into mice. If one assumes that 1000 Tani units are equivalent to 10 μg of crystalline tetrodotoxin (c f. Kao, 1966), then the ovaries of the following fish contained less than 0.2 μg of tetrodotoxin per gram: *Lagocephalus inermis, Lagocephalus spadiceus, Liosaccus cutaneus, Diodon halocanthus,* and *Chilomycterus affinis.* Several studies have been made of the toxicity of organs of the puffers of the Atlantic and Gulf coasts of the United States. Larson *et al.* (1960) found that the gonads of the northern puffer, *Sphaeroides maculatus,* * and the checkered puffer, *S. testudineus,* taken off Florida were frequently, but not invariably, toxic when injected into animals. The toxin was not identified, but the symptoms resembled those produced by tetrodotoxin. Calculations from their data (Lalone *et al.,* 1963) show that if the toxin is indeed tetrodotoxin the ovaries may contain about 0.06 μg/g. Lynch *et al.* (1967), using methods that should detect about that amount of toxin, could not show toxicity in any tissues of *S. maculatus* caught off New Jersey during May to July. When ovarian extracts were concentrated they obtained about

---

*In a recent publication Shipp and Yerger (1969) claim that the range of *S. maculatus* extends only as far south as Jacksonville, Florida, while that of *S. nephelus* extends down the east coast of Florida and into the Gulf of Mexico. This suggests that the puffers studied by Larson *et al.* (1960) were the latter species, but Burklew and Morton (1971) found *S. nephelus* from the Gulf coast of Florida to be nontoxic.

0.005 μg/gm ovary, although large losses must have occurred. We found that ovaries of S. *maculatus* taken off Coney Island in September contained toxicity equivalent to about 0.05 μg/gm of tetrodotoxin (Fuhrman *et al.*, 1969).

Larson *et al.* (1960) reported that the ovaries of *Lagocephalus laevigatus* and *Chilomycterus schoepfi* from Florida were not toxic, nor were two species of fish of the genus *Lactophrys* (family Ostraciontidae). Burklew and Morton (1971) reported that the viscera of *Sphaeroides spengleri* were toxic when injected into mice, but the toxicity of the ovaries was not reported separately. Viscera of S. *nephelus* and S. *dorsalis* from the Gulf coast of Florida were not toxic (Burklew and Morton, 1971).

C. Distribution of Tetrodotoxin in Organs

In both puffer fish and newts, tetrodotoxin is found in very high concentration in the eggs and ovaries, (Miura and Takesaki, 1890), and in variable but lower concentrations in the liver and skin, depending upon the species and the season of the year. The data in Table II illustrate the distribution of the toxin in some representative species of puffer fish. The first five species are important food fish in Japan. It is clear that the ovaries of all these species of *Fugu* contain large amounts of toxin. As the ova mature and the ovaries increase in size during the fall and winter, not only does the total

TABLE II
Distribution of Tetrodotoxin in the Organs of Female Fish
(in micrograms per gram fresh weight)[a]

	Ovary	Liver	Skin	Intestine	Muscle
Fugu paradalis	200	1000	100	40	1
Fugu vermicularis vermicularis	400	200	100	40	4
Fugu vermicularis porphyreus	400	200	20	40	1
Fugu rubripes rubripes	100	100	10	20	< 0.2
Fugu ocellatus obscurus	1000	40	20	40	< 0.2
Fugu niphobles	400	1000	40	400	4
Lagocephalus inernus	0.4	1	< 0.2	0.4	0.4

[a]From Tani (1945) assuming 100 units = 1 μg tetrodotoxin.

TABLE III
Seasonal Variation of Tetrodotoxin in the Ovaries of *Fugu rubripes rubripes*[a]

Month	Ovary mean weight (gm)	Tetrodotoxin in ovary (μg/gm)	Tetrodotoxin in ovary (μg/ovary)
October	5	0.33	2
November	7	0.56	4
December	126	16.8	2113
January	132	19.0	2508
February	260	18.6	4836
March	567	7.0	3941
April	567	14.1	7882
May	155	15.7	2432
June	54	12.4	670

[a]Calculated from Tani (1945), assuming 100 units = 1 μg tetrodotoxin.

quantity of toxin in the organ increase, but the eggs contain more toxin per gram (Table III). The concentration of toxin in the liver also increases at the same time. When fertilized eggs of *Fugu niphobles* were examined for toxicity, it was found that the amount of toxin remained unchanged during the early stages of development, but decreased by about 50% at the time of hatching (Suyama and Uno, 1957–1958). It is possible that the decrease resulted from diffusion of the toxin following destruction of the egg casing.

D. CHEMISTRY OF TETRODOTOXIN

Crystalline tetrodotoxin has been prepared from the ovaries of several species of puffers: *Fugu rubripes* (Yokoo, 1950; Nagai, 1956), *Fugu vermicularis* (Kakisawa *et al.*, 1959), and *F. stictonotus* (Arakawa, 1956), and from the eggs and embryos of the newt, *Taricha torosa* (Brown and Mosher, 1963). The chemical and pharmacological properties of tetrodotoxin from the various sources mentioned, and from puffer fish liver, are identical (Saito, 1961; Buchwald *et al.*, 1964).

Although crystalline tetrodotoxin was isolated in 1950, the determination of the structure proved to be extraordinarily difficult

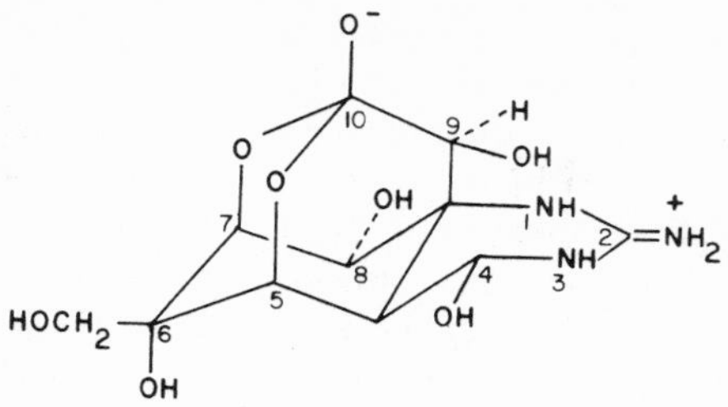

Fig. 2. Tetrodotoxin.

in spite of the fact that ample supplies of material were available. The molecular formula is $C_{11}H_{17}N_3O_8$, and the structure is shown in Fig. 2. The pKa is 8.7. The crystalline toxin is practically insoluble in water and in the usual organic solvents. Less pure material is easily soluble in water, and the crystalline toxin may be dissolved in weak acid. The structure of tetrodotoxin presents several unusual features which may contribute to its unusually interesting pharmacological properties. The cyclic hemilactal structure is unknown in any other natural or synthetic compound. The toxin exists in solution as a zwitterion with a guanidinium cation and an hemilactal anion. Even relatively small alterations in the chemical structure abolish the pharmacological activity (Deguchi, 1967). More details of the chemistry of tetrodotoxin are given by Mosher et al. (1964), Tsuda (1966), and Woodward (1964).

The stability of tetrodotoxin to heating in aqueous solutions is markedly dependent upon the pH of the solution. At about pH 7 little or no inactivation occurs during boiling in water for 30–60 minutes (Tahara, 1910; Van Wagtendonk et al., 1942; Shirota et al., 1952) or autoclaving for 1 hour at 120°C. (Horsburgh et al., 1940). The toxin can be partially or completely inactivated by heating in acid solutions at pH 4 or below (Waterfield and Evans, 1972), or in alkaline solutions at pH 9 or above; inactivation occurs more readily in alkaline than in acid solutions (Van Wagtendonk et al., 1942; Yokoo, 1950; Shirota et al., 1952). It is to be expected that little toxin would be inactivated in fish prepared by ordinary cooking. The usual commercial canning method applied to puffer fish in one-half pound tins inactivated some, but not all, of the toxin in the tissues (Halstead and Bunker, 1953).

E. Tetrodotoxin Poisoning in Man

In Japan certain species of puffer fish, especially *Fugu rubripes rubripes (Torafugu)* (Fig. 1A) are highly esteemed as food. Since the amount of tetrodotoxin in the muscle is quite low, poisoning most frequently occurs from contamination of the edible parts of the fish with ovaries or liver, or ingestion of these internal organs by uninformed people. Ogura (1958) summarized the statistics on tetrodotoxin poisoning in Japan since 1886. The number of deaths has remained fairly constant at about 100 per year over a period of 70 years. In 1958 there were 289 cases of poisoning with a mortality of 60.9%, and in 1959 there were 211 cases of poisoning with a mortality of 56% (Tsuda, 1966). In an effort to reduce human poisoning various control measures have been introduced. These vary with the locality, and range from total prohibition of the sale of puffer fish, through removal of the viscera in the fish market accompanied by thorough washing of the edible portion, to licensing of cooks authorized to prepare these fish in special restaurants (cf. Halstead, 1967). Control is difficult, however, for several reasons. Many fish never pass through the fish markets, and some are consumed by people who cannot identify the poisonous organs (ovaries and liver). Puffers are considered to be especially delicious in the winter, at the time when the concentration of tetrodotoxin in the ovaries and liver is highest; in summer, when they are relatively nontoxic, they are not so highly esteemed as food (Tsuda, 1966). In addition, many orientals consider a slight numbness of the lips and tongue and a sensation of warmth (clearly signs of mild tetrodotoxin intoxication) to be one of the most enjoyable aspects of eating puffer fish. Obviously, the amount of toxin must be very carefully controlled, since tetrodotoxin has one of the steepest dose–response curves known (Section IIF).

In certain areas of Japan, the roe of puffer fish is pickled in salt and rice bran and aged for 3 to 4 years before being eaten (Migita and Hashimoto, 1951). The roe is taken from poisonous species, but the long storage period is sufficient for most of the toxin to be destroyed.

In intoxication by tetrodotoxin in man, toxic signs and symptoms generally appear in 30–60 minutes, but occasionally sooner.

According to Professor Fukuda (cf. Ogura, 1971), the following stages may be recognized:

1. Numbness of the lips, tongue, and often of fingers. Nausea, vomiting, and anxiety.

2. Numbness becomes more marked. Muscular paralysis of extremities without loss of tendon reflexes.

3. Ataxia and motor incoordination, becoming more severe. Paralysis develops. Consciousness is present, but speaking difficult because of paralysis.

4. Consciousness lost. Death from respiratory paralysis.

According to Ogura (1971), prognosis is unfavorable if toxic signs develop rapidly, if vomiting is severe, or if the signs listed above in the third and fourth categories develop. There is no antidote. Treatment consists of efforts to remove tetrodotoxin from the gastrointestinal tract (gastric lavage, emesis, and catharsis), to support respiration (artificial respiration is important and effective), and to prevent circulatory failure. There is no antiserum, since tetrodotoxin is not antigenic. The fatal oral dose in man is estimated to be equivalent to about 1–2 mg of crystalline tetrodotoxin (cf. Tani, 1945; Evans, 1969). This amount might be contained in as little as a gram or so of ovary from a highly toxic species such as *Fugu oscellatus obscurus* during the winter months, but usually a dose of 10 gm or more of roe would be required to produce fatal poisoning.

Most cases of tetrodotoxin poisoning occur in Japan because of the presence there of highly toxic puffer fish and the common use of these fish as food. Occasionally, however, fatal poisoning occurs elsewhere such as Florida from *Sphaeroides maculatus*(Fig. 1C) (Benson, 1956), Egypt from *Arothron hispidus* (Fig. 1D) (Abdallah and Kamel, 1970), and India (Jones, 1956).

F. PHARMACOLOGY OF TETRODOTOXIN

1. Bioassay

There are no specific chemical methods available for the detection of tetrodotoxin, and therefore it is necessary to rely on a bioassay. In the early studies of tetrodotoxin from newt eggs it was found that there was approximately an exponential relationship between the time required for death after subcutaneous injection into a mouse and the dose (Horsburgh *et al.*, 1940). More recently (Wakely *et al.*, 1966) intraperitoneal injection was used. The specificity of the method was greatly enhanced by dialysis of weakly acidic crude tissue extracts against water, and concentration of the aqueous solution before injection (cf. Wakely *et al.*, 1966). Ogura (1958b) proposed a similar method for estimating the toxicity of puffer fish, and showed with crystalline tetrodotoxin that there was an exponential relationship between time required to produce death and dose. By adjusting the dose to give a death time between 1 and 15 minutes, the method is more rapid and convenient than estimation of the LD_{50} by conventional methods. The method is sufficiently sensitive to detect about 0.5 μg tetrodotoxin. McFarren (1967) showed that tetrodotoxin and saxitoxin (from dinoflagellates occurring in shellfish) could be differentiated from ciguatoxin by an assay of this kind. Other assay methods for tetrodotoxin are discussed by Kao (1966). See Chapter 4 for more detailed discussion of saxitoxin and ciguatoxin.

2. *Effects in Experimental Animals.*

All vertebrate animals so far studied, with the exception of those that produce tetrodotoxin (fish of the order Tetraodontiformes and newts of the family Salamandridae) are affected by tetrodotoxin (Ishihara, 1919; Kao and Fuhrman, 1967). In mice the relationship between dose and response is extremely steep: by intraperitoneal injection the minimum lethal dose was 8 μg/kg, while a dose of 12 μg/kg killed all the animals; the LD_{50} estimated graphically was 10 μg/kg (Kao and Fuhrman, 1963). Ogura (cf. Ogura 1971) found the LD_{50} by intraperitoneal injection into mice to be 11 μg/kg; he also lists median lethal doses for several other experimental animals by different routes of administration. Orally the LD_{50} is approximately 20 times that by intraperitoneal or intravenous administration.

In experimental animals, the intravenous administration of doses of 1–5 μg/kg of crystalline tetrodotoxin produced a rapid weakening of muscular contraction, depression of respiration, and profound hypotension. These effects have been extensively investigated by a variety of methods and good reviews of the details of the pharmacology have been published (Kao, 1966; Evans, 1969; Ogura, 1971). These should be consulted for details and only a brief summary will be given here.

As long ago as 1919 Ishihara showed that propagated action potentials are blocked by tetrodotoxin in the nerves of intact animals. The details of this blockage are now well known (see section IIE3). In addition to an effect on axonal conduction, the toxin also has a direct blocking effect on skeletal muscle fibers. Thus, one of the most dramaic effects of the toxin when administered to unanesthetized animals is a weakening of voluntary muscles that is seen as a wobbling gait followed by paralysis. Although contraction of skeletal muscles elicited by indirect stimuli fails before that elicited directly, it can be shown that this is due to a more rapid effect of the toxin on the nerve than on the muscle, and not to an action of the toxin on neuromuscular transmission (cf. Kao and Fuhrman, 1963; Kao, 1966). In anesthetized cats a dose of 1 μg/kg intravenously produces hypotension and depression of respiration. With larger doses (4–5 μg/kg) respiration fails completely, but the animal can be maintained by artificial respiration. For many years it had been thought, particularly by Japanese pharmacologists, that these effects were produced predominantly by a depressant effect of tetrodotoxin on the central medullary centers. It is now clear, chiefly from the work of Kao and his collaborators, that the hypotension and respiratory depression can be accounted for by a peripheral action of the toxin. Kao *et al.* (1967) showed, by cross-perfusion experiments, that tetrodotoxin applied to the brain alone produced neither hypotension nor respiratory depression, while tetrodotoxin applied to the body alone produced profound hypotension and respiratory depression. It could be shown that the hypotension produced by low doses of tetrodotoxin resulted from a direct relaxing effect of the toxin on vascular smooth muscle, while that produced by higher doses involved release of vasomotor tone as well (Kao and Fuhrman, 1963; Lipsius *et al.*, 1968; Kao *et al.*, 1971).

Tetrodotoxin induces vomiting in dogs, cats and man in doses of the order of 1 μg/kg when injected intravenously (Hayamo and

Ogura, 1963). The emetic effect is not apparent in anesthetized animals.

3. Mechanism of Action.

The availability of crystalline tetrodotoxin provided neurophysiologists with a powerful tool for investigation of excitable membranes of nerve and muscle. This is because tetrodotoxin blocks conduction by a highly specific effect on the movement of sodium ions—and not of potassium ions—across cell membranes.

Nerve and muscle fibers are surrounded by a membrane which makes possible widely different ionic compositions of the fluids inside and outside the membranes. The inside is electrically negative to the outside by about 70 mV, and contains a relatively high concentration of potassium and relatively little sodium and chloride. In the resting state the membrane is permeable to potassium and chloride ions, but not to sodium ions. The basis of excitation consists of a series of self-limiting changes in permeability of the membrane to sodium and potassium ions. A stimulus of any kind results in a sudden, transient increase in the permeability of the membrane to sodium ions. This is followed by a more prolonged increase in permeability to potassium ions. The result of these changes in permeability is the action potential of nerve or muscle. Following the action potential the original ionic composition is restored, in part through operation of an active transport of sodium ions outward through the membrane. Local anesthetics such as procaine block the action potential by affecting both phases of ionic movements through the membrane—that is, by blocking movement of both potassium and sodium ions. This prevents the action potential from developing and thus blocks conduction in nerve axons. Tetrodotoxin, however, selectively blocks the early transient increase in permeability of the membrane to sodium ions without affecting the permeability to potassium ions (Narahashi et al., 1964; Takata et al., 1966). This effect is shown in Fig. 3, and it is this highly selective action that has made tetrodotoxin such a useful tool in investigation of the events in nerve and muscle during excitation. It is remarkable that this effect is also produced by one other toxin whose structure differs significantly from that of tetrodo-

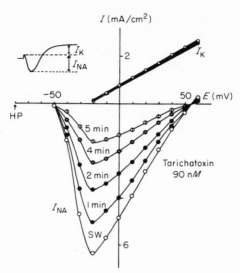

Fig. 3. Sodium and potassium current-voltage relationships observed by voltage-clamp measurements on a giant axon of the lobster at various times after application of 90 nM tetrodotoxin. HP is the holding potential. The line marked SW is the control relationship in sea water without toxin. The experiment was done with tetrodotoxin isolated from eggs of the newt, *Taricha torosa*, then designated tarichatoxin but now known to be identical to that from the puffer fish. The figure shows that tetrodotoxin selectively depresses the early transient inward current (sodium current, I_{Na}) while leaving unaffected the late outward current (potassium current, I_K). From Takata *et al.* (1966).

toxin: saxitoxin, the paralytic shellfish poison produced by dino-flagellates. Several recent reviews should be consulted for the details of the action of these toxins (Moore and Narahashi, 1967; Hille, 1971; Dettbarn, 1971; Kao, 1972; Narahashi, 1972; Evans, 1972).

III. Lipoprotein Toxins

The toxins from the eggs of two marine fish, the northern blenny of Japan and the cabezon of western North America, are

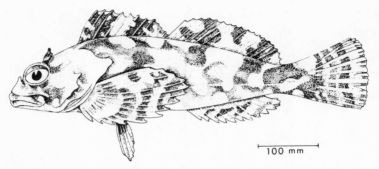

Fig. 4. The cabezon, *Scorpaenichthys marmoratus* (Ayers).

lipoproteins that produce, several hours after ingestion, a severe
illness that includes headache, diarrhea, vomiting, chest pain, and
sometimes coma and death. The toxins from the eggs of the two
fish appear to be chemically similar.

A. CABEZON ROE TOXIN

The cabezon, or marbled sculpin, *Scorpaenichthys marmoratus*
(Ayers) (Order Perciformes, Family Cottidae) (Fig. 4) is the largest
of the North American sculpins and is a common fish on the Pacific
Coast from Mexico to Alaska. While it is of minor commercial importance as a food fish, it is taken in large numbers by sport fisher-
men (O'Connell, 1953). The flesh is edible, although somewhat
coarse, but it is sometimes rejected by the unsophisticated buyer
because it is frequently light blue or green in color before cooking.
The roe, however, is poisonous.

1. History and General Effects

The first recorded instance of poisoning from eating cabezon
roe occurred in 1923 when the ichthylologist Carl Hubbs and his
wife became ill after eating the roe of a cabezon taken at Point
Lobos, California. Hubb's experience is apparently the origin of

statements by Walford (1931) and Schultz (1938) that cabezon roe is poisonous. Sommer demonstrated a slow-acting toxin in the eggs of a cottid fish from California (unidentified, but probably cabezon) that produced macroscopic changes in the liver (Sommer and Meyer, 1937). It was not until the publication by Hubbs and Wick (1951) that clear evidence of the toxicity of cabezon eggs appeared in the literature. They recounted the earlier experience of the senior author and presented evidence that ground cabezon roe administered orally produced illness and death in mice and guinea pigs. Pillsbury (1957) observed that in British Columbia the eggs of the cabezon were avoided by birds, mink, and raccoons that readily ate the eggs of other fishes.

The symptoms of poisoning by cabezon eggs appear a few hours after eating them. Hubbs described them as "rapidly alternating chills and fever with frequent vomiting and diarrhea" (Hubbs and Wick, 1951). Russell (1965, and personal communication) observed two cases and described the symptoms as follows: "The poisoning is characterized by the rapid onset of nausea, vomiting and epigastric distress. Diarrhea, dryness in the mouth, thirst, tinnitus, and malaise sometimes occur. In the more severe cases, syncopy, respiratory distress, chest pain, convulsions, and coma may ensue. Complete recovery usually occurs within a few days."

We have investigated the effects of cabezon roe toxin in experimental animals (Fuhrman *et al.,* 1969, 1970). Roe were collected from many fish over a period of several years and all samples were found to be toxic. Simple saline extracts prepared by homogenizing and centrifuging the eggs in 0.9% NaCl were used for many experiments. These extracts, administered either orally or intraperitoneally, caused a reproducible sequence of events in mice and rats. With surely lethal doses the animals sought the corners of the cages and exhibited ruffled fur after about 12 hours. They then became inactive, sometimes with diarrhea and nasal discharge, and then became comatose and died in 15–24 hours. The lethal dose was about 4 gm dry roe/kg administered orally and about 2 gm dry roe/kg administered intraperitoneally. Similar aqueous extracts of liver, testes, and spent ovaries were not toxic in doses about four times this great. It was established that the toxicity of the roe was not caused by contaminating microorganisms.

2. Chemistry

The toxin from cabezon eggs is not dialyzable through Visking tubing. The toxicity of aqueous extracts is destroyed at 95°C for 10 minutes, and dried preparations of the toxin were inactivated after a few weeks at room temperature. Some purification could be obtained by precipitation of the toxin from $0.1M$ NaCl solution with ammonium sulfate or alcohol. The toxin was also precipitated by dilution with large volumes of distilled water. Approximately tenfold purification of the toxin was achieved by two different methods (Fuhrman *et al.*, 1969). In one the toxin was precipitated from $0.14M$ NaCl by reducing the pH to 4.25. The toxic precipitate was dissolved in $0.14M$ NaCl at pH 6.9 and the toxin was again precipitated by increasing the sodium chloride concentration to 180 gm/liter. The toxic material had an LD_{50} by intraperitoneal injection into mice of 150 mg/kg and contained 6.70% N and 0.85% P. In the other method the toxin was purified on polyacrylamide gel. The most toxic fractions had an LD_{50} of 200 mg/kg and contained 11.6% N and 0.61% P. Both preparations were toxic when administered orally to mice. The toxin purified by column chromatography contained 1.4% lipid extractable with cold chloroform. Both preparations of toxin, although impure, appear to be lipoproteins or complexes in which a toxin is bound to such a molecule.

3. Pharmacology

The toxin from cabezon roe is not hemolytic, or proteolytic. It does not increase vascular permeability and has no effect on contraction of intestinal or vascular smooth muscle, on conduction in frog sciatic nerve, or on circulatory dynamics within 8 hours after injection (Fuhrman *et al.*, 1969). However, this toxin did inhibit the growth of mouse fibroblasts grown in tissue culture in reasonable concentrations of about 6 mouse lethal doses per liter, and this effect was dependent on concentration (Fuhrman *et al.*, 1970). The pathological effects (see following Section 4) suggested that cabezon roe toxin might affect the numbers and kinds of white blood cells in the peripheral circulation. This was found to be the case (Fuhrman *et al.*, 1970). Intraperitoneal injection of sterile saline solutions of the toxin into mice increased the concentration of total white blood cells at 14 and 20 hours after injection, and at the same time decreased the number of mononucleated cells per milliliter blood at the same time periods. These changes probably reflect the changes produced by the toxin in the liver and spleen (see Section IIA4).

4. Pathology

The pathological effects of various doses of saline extracts of cabezon roe were studied in mice at different times after injection by A. M. Saunders and F. A. Fuhrman (unpublished, 1968). Within 20–30 hours after intraperitoneal injection of approximately one median lethal dose the livers of these mice contained focal necroses of groups of 4 to 10 cells, around which polymorphonuclear neutrophils were aggregated. At the same time, and earlier, there was a striking depletion of lymphocytes from the red pulp of the spleen. The germinal follicles appeared smaller with degenerating cells at the edges. In splenectomized mice the focal necrosis of the liver was much reduced, but the mice died with the usual sequence of signs. The major pathological effect of cabezon roe thus appears to be a rapid depletion of lymphocytes in the spleen, with secondary necrosis of the liver. The cause of death could not be established, and occurred in splenectomized animals with minimal hepatic necrosis.

B. BLENNY ROE TOXIN: LIPOSTICHAERIN

The northern blenny, *Stichaeus grigorjewi* Herzenstein (formerly *Dinogunellus grigorjewi*) (Order Perciformes, Family Stichaeidae)

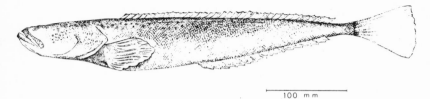

100 mm

Fig. 5. The Japanese northern blenny, *Stichaeus grigorjewi* (Herzenstein).

(Figure 5), is widely distributed in the sea of northern Japan and is used there as a source of food.

1. History and General Effects

It is said that in Hokkaido the roe has been long known to be toxic. Following a series of poisonings in 1952–1953, Takayanagi *et al.* (1953) successfully reproduced the symptoms of poisoning in human subjects and found that 20–30 gm of the raw roe were sufficient to produce the symptoms.

Two cases of poisoning are described by Asano and Itoh (1962). The symptoms of poisoning appeared several hours after eating the roe and consisted of headache, diarrhea, nausea and vomiting, abdominal pain, a sensation of constriction in the chest, dizziness, and (in one patient) hypotension, coma, and death about 23 hours after first eating the roe.

2. Chemistry

The true toxin in blenny roe that is responsible for poisoning in man must be one that is effective when administered orally to animals. Two groups of Japanese workers fractionated the roe by several different methods and obtained a number of lipid and lipoprotein preparations that were toxic when administered intraperitoneally to mice, but were not toxic when administered orally, It must be emphasized that these toxic fractions, although of chemical and pharmacological interest, cannot include the native toxin from the roe. The first preparation that was toxic by oral administration was obtained by Asano and Itoh (1966) using a method of extraction with organic solvents based on that of Thiele. Only one fraction, the ethanol insoluble lipid fraction, was toxic orally, and this was designated δ-lipostichaerin.* It was also toxic when administered intraperitoneally. The best preparations con-

---

*The terminology of the lipostichaerins is analogous to that of the lipovitellins (cf. Bernardi and Cook, 1960). Three lipostichaerins of varying densities were fractionated by Asano and Itoh (1966) and were designated α-, β-, and γ-lipostichaerin. The lipoprotein isolated by solvent fractionation was designated δ-lipostichaerin.

tained about 6% N and 2.1% P, amino acids, glycerol, and fatty acids. The authors consider it to be a lipoprotein or lipopeptide.

Several years earlier Asano and Itoh (1962) and Sakai *et al.* (1962) obtained lipoprotein fractions from blenny roe and showed that these were toxic intraperitoneally (no indication of oral toxicity was published). Asano (1964) reported the preparation of two complex lipids from the roe, both of which were toxic by intra-peritoneal administration. Hatano *et al.* (1964) prepared several fractions that were toxic intraperitoneally, the best of which had a toxicity of about 260 mg/kg and appeared to be a complex lipo-protein. Asano and Itoh (1966) fractionated the roe by centrifu-gation and obtained three lipoproteins of varying density, all of which were toxic intraperitoneally but not orally. The lipid moieties of two of these were also toxic intraperitoneally but not orally. Several of these fractions were well characterized chemically by determination of amino acid and fatty acid constituents, but the relationship of these substances to the true oral toxin is obscure.

More recently Hatano (1970a) reported the purification by ammonium sulfate precipitation of a lipoprotein that resembled the lipostichaerin of Asano and Itoh (1966), and which he also designated lipostichaerin. This lipostichaerin appears to have the properties of the true blenny roe toxin. It, as well as its lipid moiety, were toxic intraperitoneally, and both produced pathological effects in animals when administered orally in sublethal doses (Hatano, 1971b). Unfortunately, no quantitative data on oral toxicity of the lipostichaerin were given. Dr. Hatano has informed me (M. Hatano, personal communication, 1972) however, that the lipostichaerin was lethal to rats when administered orally in doses of about 300 mg/kg or greater. This lipostichaerin is a high-density lipoprotein containing 12.16% N and 0.88% P (Hatano, 1970b). The lipid moiety of this lipostichaerin, a phospholipid, was toxic by intraperitoneal injection (Hatano, 1971a). The phospholipid was obtained in a highly purified form (Hatano, 1971d). It contained 7.33% N and 2.68% P, peptides containing aspartic acid and glycine, and fatty acids. The lipoprotein (lipostichaerin), was chromatographically homogeneous (Hatano, 1971c). It was a high density lipoprotein with a molecular weight of 4×10^5, containing 12.16% N and 0.88% P. The LD_{50} by intraperitoneal injection was

180 mg/kg, but the oral toxicity was not given. No comparable toxic material could be prepared from muscle or sperm of the blenny.

In summary, lipoproteins from the roe of the northern blenny *Stichaeus grigorjewi* that have been designated lipostichaerins have been obtained by Asano and Itoh (1966) and Hatano (1970a). These lipoproteins meet the criteria of the true toxin of the roe. Since the lipid moiety of these lipoproteins is also toxic, it is probable that the toxicity of the native lipostichaerin is attributable to that of the lipid fraction (M. Hatano, personal communication, 1972).

3. Pharmacology and Pathology

The δ-lipostichaerin of Asano and Itoh (1966) was lethal when administered orally to rats in doses of 4–6 gm/kg. No mention is made of the symptoms produced. The lipostichaerin of Hatano (1971c) was reported to produce the following sequence of symptoms when injected intraperitoneally into mice in a dose of 1.1 gm/kg: after 10–13 hours dullness of the hair coat and pilo-erection; photophobia; after 20–24 hours staggering gait and paralysis followed by loss of reflexes and convulsions and death (Hatano, 1971a).

Asano and Itoh (1962) showed that the toxic lipoprotein from blenny roe, when injected intraperitoneally, produced increased amounts of fat in the livers. The fat could be demonstrated both histologically and chemically. Similar changes were produced by several toxic lipids (Asano and Itoh, 1962; Asano, 1964). Hatano (1971a) injected lipostichaerin and the toxic phospholipid intra-peritoneally and observed cloudy swelling of the liver and enlarge-ment of the spleen and kidney with the lipostichaerin, and hemorrhage of the spleen and kidney with the phospholipid.

A more comprehensive study of the effects of lipostichaerin and the toxic phospholipid from blenny roe has been published re-cently by Hatano (1971b). The substances were administered both orally and intraperitoneally to rats, and 6 hours later the animals were sacrificed. Both toxic substances produced decreases in the concentration of total lipids, neutral lipids, and cholesterol in the plasma. The effects were more marked after intraperitoneal than oral administration. No significant changes occurred in hematocrit, total protein or various globulin fractions, glucose, bilirubin, Na, or K. Both toxic fractions also increased serum glutamic–oxalacetic transaminase (GOT), serum glutamic–pyruvic transaminase (GPT), serum lactic dehydrogenase and amylase, while they had no effect on alkaline phosphatase and cholinesterase. The effects were more marked following intraperitoneal than oral administration. At autopsy (6 hours after administration) no changes were seen in parenchymal organs after administration of the lipostichaerin by either route, but the liver was enlarged and the intestine congested after administration of the toxic phospholipid.

These studies of the effects of toxic fractions of blenny roe in animals indicate that both lipostichaerin and the toxic phospholipid produce pathological changes in the liver and may affect the spleen, kidney, pancreas, and intestines. Of particular significance is the observation that serum transaminases and serum lactic dehydrogenase increase within 6 hours after administration of the toxins. These enzymes are normally intracellular and are released into the serum following damage to parenchymal cells of the liver, or to cells of other tissues. Increased serum amylase is usually associated with pancreatitis, and may indicate an action of these toxins on that organ as well.

IV. Toxins from Eggs of Cyprinid Fishes, Pikes, and Gars

The eggs of a number of freshwater fishes, mostly members of the carp family (Cyprinidae), but also of pikes and gars, produce symptoms of mild to severe gastroenteritis when eaten. So little is known about these toxins that evidence for their chemical similarity does not exist, but the symptomology of poisoning suggests that they are related.

A. CYPRINIDAE

The family Cyprinidae (Order Cypriniformes) includes a large number of fish such as carps and minnows, a few of which are known to have poisonous roe.

1. Barbus (Barbel, Barbe, Barbeau, Barbo)

Two species of barbel are common in the rivers of Europe: *Barbus barbus* (Linnaeus) in northern and central Europe, and *Barbus meridionalis* (Risso) in the Mediterranean region. Ingestion of the eggs of either species produces diarrhea, nausea, and vomiting within a few hours after ingestion. The intoxication has been called "Barbencholera" because of the similarity of symptoms to those of true cholera.

The older literature contains many descriptions of poisoning from eating barbel eggs in addition to the experimental demonstration of toxicity by Antonio Gazio mentioned in the introduction. Meyer-Ahrens (1855) cites some 18 references to poisoning from barbel eggs, and gives detailed accounts of several episodes of poisoning. Others have been described by von Franque (1858) and Münchmeyer (1875). The latter, for example, relates that in the evening he was called to the home of a teacher whom he found in an alarming condition:

> er hatte sich 5-mal hintereinander in heftigster Weise erbrochen, ebenso rasch folgten sich gleichzeitig unter starken Leibschmerzen 9–10 diarrhoische Stuhlentleerungen von dunkelgrüner Farbe; die Gesichtszüge waren bleich und eingefallen, die Pupillen etwas erweitert, der Puls nur schwach fühlbar, die allgemeine Prostration sehr ausgesprochen; auserdem Klagen über ein sehr unangenehmes Gefühl im Schlunde, jedoch keine Schlingbeschwerden.

The patient rapidly recovered. Two days later, however, he experienced the same symptoms again. On both days he had eaten a barbel, cooked with its roe, for lunch.

From the uniformity of the symptoms reported, and the multiplicity of the instances of poisoning it is clear that these eggs must contain a toxin, and that these poisonings cannot be attributed to spoilage. Nevertheless, barbel roe is not always toxic and is reputed to be most poisonous in spring and early summer when the eggs become mature. The principal symptoms (cf. Meyer-Ahrens, 1855; McCrudden, 1921) include abdominal distention and pain beginning a few hours after eating the roe, nausea, stomach ache, cold extremities, malaise, vomiting, and diarrhea. No fatal cases have been reported.

McCrudden (1911, 1921) reported the results of a series of chemical and pharmacological experiments designed to isolate and identify the nature of the toxic material in the eggs of barbel and pike (see below). He does not record any experiment in which the oral toxicity of barbel roe was tested. He found, however, that a partially purified aqueous solution of dried barbel roe produced dyspnea and death from respiratory failure when injected into rabbits in doses equivalent to 0.65–0.75 gm/kg dry roe. Whatever the nature of the toxic material in this crude extract, it is doubtful that it bears any relationship to the toxin present in fresh roe responsible for the symptoms described above.

2. Tinca (Tench, Schleibe, Tanche)

The eggs of the tench, *Tinca tinca* (Linnaeus) are frequently listed as poisonous. In a sixteenth century treatise on veterinary medicine by Laurentii Rusii the eggs of the tench (as well as those of the barbel) were recommended for the purging of horses. This observation has been repeated in a number of well-known reviews and monographs on animal toxins (Meyer-Ahrens, 1855; Phisalix, 1922; Pawlowsky, 1927; Hiyama, 1950). There does not appear to be any experimental confirmation of the statement or any case reports of poisoning in man.

3. Abramis (Breme, Brachsen, Bley, Brax)

The roe of the bream *Abramis brama* (Linnaeus) has been reported to be poisonous and similar to the roe of the barbel (Pawlowsky, 1927). However, Meyer-Ahrens (1855) mentions that the eggs are considered poisonous on the Volga, but not in France and Germany. There does not appear to be any case reports of poisoning or experimental work on these eggs, and it appears doubtful that they are uniformly poisonous.

4. Schizothorax (Snow Trout, Gebirgsbarbe)

Schizothorax intermedius (McClelland), a fine-scaled carp is native to central Asia. Pawlowsky (1927) quotes a passage attributed to Kuschelevsky from Berg's (1905) *Fische von Turkestan:*

> The roe is coarse-grained, yellowish-red in color, resembling that of pike, is very tasty, but highly poisonous, as I observed many times in Fergana and in the Kirghiz Steppes. When the fish were caught

usually the roe and entrails were removed and discarded on the bank
of the stream; even the crows did not touch them, though it is well
known that these birds are voracious and not particular in choice of
food. When an uknowing bird ate the roe, he died immediately, as I
have observed in the Kirghiz Steppes.

Knox (1888) fed the roe of *S. argentatus* Kessler that had been
preserved in alcohol and then thoroughly washed, to mice. Death
was reported to have occurred about 30 hours later.

B. PIKE

The pike, *Esox lucius* (Linnaeus) (called Hecht, brochet), is a very
large fish found in many of the rivers and lakes of Europe. Since
the sixteenth century various authors have reported the eggs to be
poisonous, and to produce gastrointestinal symptoms similar to
those produced by the eggs of the barbel (see Meyer-Ahrens, 1855;
Phisalix, 1922; Pawlowsky, 1927; Romano, 1940). The effect, however, appears to be less consistent and not so well documented as
for barbel eggs. Chevallier and Duchesne (1851) consider the eggs
to be poisonous only from March to September and they cite five
references to articles describing their toxicity. Certainly the eggs of
the pike were considered to be sufficiently poisonous in Germany
that McCrudden (1921), working in Faust's laboratory in
Würzburg, used them for most of his experimental work on the
chemical and pharmacological properties of barbel and pike roe.
Nevertheless, he found that 324 gm of pike roe when fed to a 6-kg
dog did not produce any symptoms at all. McCrudden (1921) prepared a protein fraction from pike roe that, when injected intravenously into rabbits, produced dyspnea, convulsions, and death in
doses of about 20–40 mg/kg. The toxin was nondialyable and heat-
labile. One may question whether this toxin bears any relationship
to that present in pike roe that produces nausea, vomiting, and
diarrhea after eating the raw roe.

C. GARS

The gar family (Lepisosteidae) comprises fewer than 10 species
which are confined to the fresh and brackish waters of North

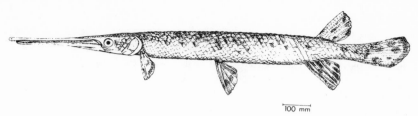

Fig. 6. The longnose gar, *Lepisosteus osseus* (Linnaeus).

America. They are distinguished by thick scales on the body, and by elongated jaws (Fig. 6).

Dr. W. Brooks of Circleville, Illinois recorded that in April, 1850, a family of five ate a freshly caught gar and its eggs for dinner (Brooks, 1851). A few hours later each of the five "felt a burning sensation in the pit of the stomach, which was soon succeeded by vomiting, purging, and cramping, in their most aggravated forms." All five persons recovered.

Several authors of reviews have stated that gar eggs are reported to be poisonous without citing specific evidence of toxicity (Coker, 1930; Luce, 1933; Taft, 1945). Luce (1933) does record, however, that "one man reported that the roe from one alligator gar killed 90 chickens." After publishing our studies on tetrodotoxin in salamander eggs (Mosher *et al.,* 1964), we received letters from several zoologists who had poisoned themselves and friends with gar roe, or with caviar prepared from gar roe. They raised the question whether gar roe might also contain tetrodotoxin. Professor George A. Moore (personal communication, 1972) writes that many years ago he and friends tried to eat the fried roe of a large longnose gar (*Lepisosteus osseus* Linnaeus) caught in a tributary to the Cimarron River in Oklahoma. The flavor was disagreeable, however, and he soon ejected the morsel of roe. Nevertheless, he and his friends experienced gastric and intestinal disturbances including nausea and diarrhea.

In a neglected abstract, Greene *et al.* (1918) describe the results of experiments in which they fed fresh gar ovaries to several kinds of experimental animals. Although the species of gar are not mentioned, they were probably *L. osseus* and *L. platostomus* (Rafinesque). Chickens fed 5–75 gm of roe in several feedings showed loss of tone and paralysis of the crop, loss of appetite, diarrhea, muscular weakness, disturbances of circulation in the comb and wattles, and depression of the central nervous system. A larger dose was fatal to chickens in 3–4 days. A dose of 5 gm was fatal to white rats, and death was preceded by general malaise, weakness, and diarrhea. Cats and dogs vomited the gar roe when it was fed to them. Chemical separation of the constitutents of the roe indicated that the toxin was in the globulin fraction.

Netsch and Witt (1962), who were apparently not aware of the experiments of Greene *et al.*, cite unpublished experiments by A. A. Case who fed eggs of the longnose gar, *L. osseus*, to chickens and found that "these eggs will make the chickens very sick in reasonably small amounts." Netsch and Witt then force-fed mice with 0.2 ml of a homogenate of the eggs of a longnose gar and found that the mice became sick, but recovered. Mice fed a similar quantity of a homogenate of the eggs of the shortnose gar, *L. platostomus*, also became sick, and one mouse died.

During our work with cabezon roe (Section IIIA), we obtained the roe of a spotted gar, *Lepisosteus productus* (Cope). Homogenates of this roe were administered to rats by stomach tube and produced, after 18–48 hours, lethargy, ruffled hair, diarrhea, and sometimes death. The LD_{50} was about 7 gm/kg, and the toxin was not dialysable through Visking tubing.

The evidence thus indicates that the eggs of several species of gars contain a large molecular weight toxin that is relatively slow-acting, and that produces gastrointestinal disturbances in man and animals. The toxin is clearly not tetrodotoxin. It resembles in its action the toxin from the eggs of the barbel and pike.

V. Miscellaneous

A. OTHER FISH REPORTED TO HAVE TOXIC ROE

Halstead and Schall (1954) reported that aqueous extracts of the roe of a creolefish, *Paranthias furcifer* Valenciennes, a member of the Serranidae family, caught off La Plata Island near the coast of

Ecuador, were toxic when injected intraperitoneally into white mice.

Aqueous extracts of the oviducts of a specimen of ratfish, *Hydrolagus colliei* Lay and Bennett, taken off Fidalgo Island, Washington in June were reported to be moderately toxic when injected intraperitoneally into white mice (Halstead and Bunker, 1952). We (F. A. Fuhrman and G. J. Fuhrman, unpublished observations, 1966) examined the toxicity of aqueous extracts of ova, oviducts, and ovaries of *Hydrolagus colliei* taken off Point Pinos, Monterey Bay, California in April and May. The fresh tissues were lyophilized and kept frozen for several weeks. Aqueous extracts were then prepared and injected into white mice. No evidence of toxicity was obtained.

It has been stated by Scott (1969) and Halstead (1967) that the roe of sturgeons (principally *Acipenser sturio* Linneaus and *Huso huso* Linnaeus) is toxic under some circumstances. I have not been able to find direct evidence for this. Certainly, caviar prepared by salting the roe of these fish is not toxic and it seems probable that any suggestion of toxicity must be attributable to bacterial contamination.

The roe of the following fishes has been stated to be poisonous but no reliable evidence for the presence of a naturally occurring toxin in these roe appears to exist: the catfishes *Selenaspis herzbergi* Bloch, *Pseudobagrus aurantiaccus* Temminck and Schlegel (Halstead, 1967; Scott, 1969) and *Argeneiosus armatus* Lacépède (Pawlowsky, 1927); the burbot *Lota lota* Linnaeus (Chevallier and Duchesne, 1851; Pawlowsky, 1927; Halstead, 1967; Scott, 1969); the perch *Perca fluviatilis* Linnaeus (Meyer-Ahrens, 1955) whose roe is said to resemble that of the barbel; the flatfish *Scophthalmus rhombus* Linnaeus (Pawlowsky, 1927).

Certain herrings and anchovies belonging to the order Clupeiformes occasionally produce a form of poisoning that has been termed clupeotoxism (Halstead, 1967). The toxic fishes appear to be restricted geographically and seasonally. According to Tybring (1886) and Kobert (1905) the tropical herring *Clupanodon thrissa* Linnaeus *(Meletta thrissa)* is considered dangerous to eat during the spawning season, and Tybring states that the roe is the most poisonous part.

B. POISONOUS EGGS OF AMPHIBIANS

The eggs of the salamander *Taricha torosa* are layed in clusters from 2 to 3 cm in diameter and containing about 20 ova each surrounded by a gelatinous material. These egg clusters contain tetrodotoxin (cf. Mosher *et al.*, 1964) and are potentially hazardous if eaten. They are frequently found in large numbers on the bottom of ponds or attached to twigs. While we do not know of any incidents of human poisoning, we have observed bass that have been poisoned by eating the egg clusters.

Licht (1967) reported the fatal poisoning of a woman and a child following ingestion of a soup made from boiled eggs of the toad *Bufo marinus*.

C. SEA URCHIN OVARIES

Jordan (1931), Phisalix (1932), Pawlowsky (1937), Halstead (1965), and others state that the ovaries of sea urchins are believed to be poisonous during the spawning season, although they are commonly consumed without harm at other seasons. The symptoms are reported to be nausea, vomiting, and diarrhea. The only experimental work on this subject appears to be that of Loisel (1903, 1904), who reported that simple extracts of the ovaries and testes of sea urchins were toxic when injected intravenously into rabbits, although only the ovarian extracts were lethal.

Acknowledgment

I wish to thank the Hopkins Marine Station for hospitality during preparation of this review, Susan Manchester for the drawings of fish used as illustrations, and Professor George A. Moore and Dr. Mutsuo Hatano for permitting me to cite unpublished work. Preparation of the article was supported in part by Grant GM16031 from the National Institutes of Health, U.S. Public Health Service.

References

Abdallah, M. M. M., and Kamel, S. (1970). *Alexandria Med. J.* **16,** 302.
Arakawa, H. (1956). *J. Chem. Soc. Jap. Pure Chem. Sect.* **77,** 1295.
Asano, M. (1964). *Tohoku J. Agr. Res.* **15,** 113.

Asano, M., and Itoh, M. (1962). *Tohoku J. Agr. Res.* **13,** 151.

Asano, M., and Itoh, M. (1966). *Tohoku J. Agr. Res.* **16,** 299.

Beaglehole, J. C. (1961). "The Journals of Captain Cook," Vol. 2, "Voyages of the Resolution and Adventure 1772–1775." Cambridge Univ. Press, London and New York.

Benson, J. (1956). *J. Forensic Sci.* **1,** 119.

Berg, L. S. (1905). *Mitth. Turkestan. Abh. K. Russ. Geogr. Gesell.* **4,** 1–261 (In Russian).

Bernardi, G., and Cook, W. H. (1960). *Biochim. Biophys. Acta* **44,** 86.

Bouder, H., Cavallo, A., and Bouder, M. J. (1962). *Bull. Inst. Oceanog. (Monaco)* **1240,** 1.

Brooks, W. (1851). *North-West. Med. Surg. J.* **3,** 437.

Brown, M. S., and Mosher, H. S. (1963). *Science* **140,** 295.

Buchwald, H. D., Durham, L., Fischer, H. G., Harada, R., Mosher, H. S., Kao, C. Y., and Fuhrman, F. A. (1964). *Science* **143,** 474.

Burklew, M. A., and Morton, R. A. (1971). *Toxicon* **9,** 205.

Chevallier, A., and Duchesne, E. A. (1851). *Ann. Hyg. Publ.* Med. *Leg.* **45,** 387; **46,** 108.

Coker, R. E. (1930). *Bull. U. S. Fish. Bur.* **45,** 141.

Deguchi, T. (1967). *Jap. J. Pharmacol.* **17,** 267.

Dettbarn, W.-D. (1971). *In* "Neuropoisons" (L. Simpson, ed.), Vol. 1, pp. 169–186. Plenum, New York.

Dolman, C. E. (1957). *Jap. J. Med. Sci. Biol.* **10,** 383.

Dolman, C. E., and Chang, H. (1953). *Can. J. Pub. Health* **44,** 231.

Dolman, C. E., Tomwich, M., Campbell, C. C. B., and Laing, W. B. (1960). *J. Infec. Dis.* **106,** 5.

Evans, M. H. (1969). *Brit. Med. Bull.* **25,** 263.

Evans, M. H. (1972). *Int. Rev. Neurobiol.* **15,** 83.

Faust, E. S. (1924). *In* "Handbuch der experimentellen Pharmakologie," Vol. 2, p. 1846. Springer-Verlag, Berlin and New York.

Fish, C. J., and Cobb, M. C. (1954). *Fish Wild. Serv. (U. S.),Res. Rep.* **36.**

Fuhrman, F. A., and Fuhrman, G. J. (1966). Unpublished Observations.

Fuhrman, F. A., Fuhrman, G. J., Dull, D. L., and Mosher, H. S. (1969). *Agr. Food Chem.* **17,** 417.

Fuhrman, F. A., Fuhrman, G. J., and Roseen, J. S. (1970). *Toxicon* **8,** 55.

Goe, D. R., and Halstead, B. W. (1953). *Calif. Fish Game* **39,** 229.

Greene, C. W., Nelson, E. E., and Baskett, E. I. (1918). *Amer. J. Physiol.* **45,** 558.

Gunnison, J. B., Cummings, J. R., and Meyer, K. F. (1936). *Proc. Soc. Exp. Biol. Med.* **35,** 278.

Halstead, B. W. (1965). "Poisonous and Venomous Marine Animals of the World," Vol. 1. U S Govt. Printing Office, Washington, D. C.

Halstead, B. W. (1967). "Poisonous and Venomous Marine Animals of the World," Vol. 2. U S Govt. Printing Office, Washington, D. C.

Halstead, B. W., and Bunker, N. C. (1952). *Copeia* **3,** 128.

Halstead, B. W., and Bunker, N. C. (1953). *Calif. Fish and Game* **39,** 219.

Halstead, B. W., and Bunker, N. C. (1954). *Zoologica (New York)* **39,** 61.

Halstead, B. W., and Schall, D. S. (1954). Unpublished experiments (cited from Halstead, 1967).

Halstead, B. W., and Schall, D. W. (1955). "Essays in the Natural Sciences in Honor of Captain Allan Hancock," p. 147. Univ. of Southern California Press, Los Angeles.

Halstead, B. W., and Schall, D. W. (1956). *Pac. Sci.* **10,** 103.

Hashimoto, Y. (1950). *Bull. Jap. Soc. Sci. Fish.* **16,** 43.

Hatano, M. (1970a). *Bull. Fac. Fish. Hokkaido Univ.* **20,** 320.

Hatano, M. (1970b). *Bull. Fac. Fish. Hokkaido Univ.* **20,** 329.

Hatano, M. (1971a). *Bull. Fac. Fish. Hokkaido Univ.* **21,** 315.

Hatano, M. (1971b). *Bull. Fac. Fish. Hokkaido Univ.* **21** 331.

Hatano, M. (1971c). *Bull. Fac. Fish. Hokkaido Univ.* **22,** 168.

Hatano, M. (1971d). *Bull. Fac. Fish. Hokkaido Univ.* **22,** 177.

Hatano, M. (1972). Personal Communication.

Hatano, M., Zama, K., Takama, K., Sakai, M., and Igarashi, H. (1964). *Bull. Fac. Fish. Hokkaido Univ.* **15,** 138.

Hayama, T., and Ogura, Y. (1963). *J. Pharmacol. Exp. Ther.* **139,** 94.

Herzberg, M. (1970). "Proceedings of the First U. S.-Japan Conference on Toxic Micro-organisms." U. S. Dept. of Interior, Washington, D. C.

Hesse, C. G. (1835). "Ueber das Gift des Barbenroges" (cited from Faust, 1924).

Hille, B. (1971). *Prog. Biophys. Mol. Biol.* **21,** 1.

Hiyama, Y. (1950). *U. S., Fish Wild. Serv. Spec. Sci. Rep.–Fish.* **25.**

Horsburgh, D. B., Tatum E. L., and Hall, V. E. (1940). *J. Pharmacol. Exp. Ther.* **68,** 284.

Hubbs, C. L., and Wick, A. N. (1951). *Calif. Fish Game* **37,** 195.

Ishihara, F. (1919). *Mitt. Med. Fak. Tokio* **20,** 376.

Jordan, E. O. (1931). "Food Poisoning and Food-borne Infection." Univ. of Chicago Press, Chicago, Illinois.

Jones, S. (1956). *Indian J. Med. Res.* **44,** 353.

Kakisawa, H., Okamura, Y., and Hirata, Y. (1959). *J. Chem. Soc. Jap.,* **80,** 1493.

Kao, C. Y. (1966). *Pharmacol. Rev.* **18,** 997.

Kao, C. Y. (1972). *Fed. Proc., Fed. Amer. Soc. Exp. Biol.* **31,** 1117.

Kao, C. Y., and Fuhrman, F. A. (1963). *J. Pharmacol. Exp. Ther.* **140,** 31.

Kao, C. Y., and Fuhrman, F. A. (1967). *Toxicon* **5,** 25.

Kao, C. Y., Suzuki, T., Kleinhaus, A. L., and Siegman, M. J. (1967). *Arch. Int. Pharmacodyn. Ther.* **165,** 438.

Kao, C. Y., Nagasawa, J., Spiegelstein, M. Y., and Cha, Y. N. (1971). *J. Pharmacol. Exp. Ther.* **178,** 110.

Knox, G. (1888). *Voenno-Med. Zh.* **161,** 399.

Kobert, R. (1905). "Ueber Giftfische und Fischgifte." Enke, Stuttgart.

Kotake, M., and Arakawa, H. (1956). *J. Inst. Polytech., Osaka City Univ., Ser. C.* **5,** 57; cited from *Chem. Abstr.* **52,** 9459 (1958).

Lalone, R. C., DeVillez, E. D., and Larson, E. (1963). *Toxicon* **1,** 159.

Larson, E., Lalone, R. C., and Rivas, L. R. (1960). *Fed. Proc., Fed. Amer. Soc. Exp. Biol.* **19,** 388.

Licht, L. E. (1967). *Toxicon* **5,** 141.

Lipsius, M., Siegman, M. J., and Kao, C. Y. (1968). *J. Pharmacol. Exp. Ther.* **164,** 60.

Loisel, G. (1903). *Compt. Rend. Soc. Biol.* **55**, 1329.
Loisel, G. (1904). *Compt. Rend. Acad. Sci.* **139**, 227.
Luce, W. W. (1933). *Ill. Natur. Hist. Surv., Bull.* **20**, 71.
Lynch, P. R., Coblentz, J. M., and Hamer, P. (1967). *Amer. J. Med. Sci.* **254**, 173.
McCrudden, F. H. (1911). *J. Chem. Soc., London, Abstr. II* **100**, 421.
McCrudden, F. H. (1921). *Naunyn-Schmiedebergs Arch. Exp. Pathol. Pharmakol.* **91**, 46.
McFarren, E. F. (1967). *In* "Animal Toxins" (F. E. Russell and P. R. Saunders, eds.) p. 85. Pergamon, Oxford.
Macht, D. I. (1942). *Heb. Med. J.* **2**, 165.
Meyer-Ahrens, K. M. (1855). *Schweiz. Z. Med. Chir. Geburtshilfe* **3**, 188; **4-5**, 269.
Migita, M., and Hashimoto, Y. (1951). *Bull. Jap. Soc. Sci. Fish.* **16**, 335.
Miura, M. and Takasaki, K. (1890). *Virchow's Arch. Pathol. Anat. Physiol.* **122**, 92.
Moore, G. A. (1972). Personal communication.
Moore, J. W., and Narahashi, T. (1967). *Fed. Proc., Fed. Amer. Soc. Exp. Biol.* **26**, 1655.
Mosher, H. S., Fuhrman, F. A., Buchwald, H. D., and Fischer, H. G. (1964). *Science* **144**, 1100.
Münchmeyer, F. (1875). *Berlin Klin. Wochenschr.* **12**, 46.
Nagai, J. (1956). *Hoppe-Seyler's Z. Physiol. Chem.* **306**, 104.
Narahashi, T. (1972). *Fed. Proc., Fed. Amer. Soc. Exp. Biol.* **31**, 1124.
Narahashi, T., Moore, J. W., and Scott, W. R. (1964). *J. Gen. Physiol.* **47**, 965.
Netsch, N. F., and Witt, A., Jr. (1962). *Trans. Amer. Fish. Soc.* **91**, 251.
Noguchi, T., and Hashimoto, Y. (1973). *Toxicon* **11**, 305.
O'Connell, C. P. (1953). "The Life History of the Cabezon," Fish Bulletin No. 93. California Dept. of Fish and Game.
Ogura, Y. (1958a). *Seitai Po Kagaku* **9**, 281.
Ogura, K. (1958b). *Annu. Rep. Inst. Food Microbiol., Chiba Univ.* **11**, 79.
Ogura, K. (1971). *In* "Neuropoisons" (L. Simpson, ed.), Vol. 1, pp. 139-158. Plenum, New York.
Pawlowsky, E. N. (1927). "Gifttiere und ihre giftigkeit." Fischer, Jena.
Pedersen, H. W. (1955). *J. Appl. Bacteriol.* **18**, 619.
Phisalix, M. (1922). "Animaux venimeux et venins." Masson, Paris.
Pillsbury, R. W. (1957). *Copeia* **3**, 251.
Rieman, H. (1969). *In* "Food-Borne Infections and Intoxications" (H. Rieman, ed.), pp. 291–328. Academic Press, New York.
Romano, S. (1940). *Natura (Milan)* **31**, 137.
Russell, F. E. (1965). *Advan. Mar. Biol.* **3**, 255.
Sakai, M., Shinano, H., Kimura, T., Eme, Y., Saka, M., and Hayashi, I. (1962). *Shokuhin Eisei Kenkyu* **2**, 53.
Saito, T. (1961). *Bull. Yamaguchi Med. Sch.* **8**, 39.
Sakaguchi, G. (1969). *In* "Food-Borne Infections and Intoxications" (H. Rieman, ed.), pp. 329–358. Academic Press, New York.
Saunders, A. M., and Fuhrman, F. A. (1968). Unpublished.
Schultz, L. P. (1938). *Nat. Geogr. Mag.* **74**, 466.

Scott, H. G. (1969). *In* "Food-Borne Infections and Intoxications" (H. Rieman, ed.), pp. 543–604. Academic Press, New York.

Schreiber, J. (1884). *Berlin Klin. Wochenschr.* **21**, 161 and 183.

Shipp, R. L., and Yerger, R. W. (1969). *Copeia* **3**, 425.

Shirota, N., Fujita, K., and Kawamura, M. (1952). *Annu. Rep. Takamine Lab.* **4**, 45.

Sommer, H., and Meyer, K. F. (1937). *Arch. Pathol.* **24**, 560.

Sugiyama, H., Bott. T. L., and Foster, E. M. (1970). *In* "Proceedings of the First U. S.—Japan Conference on Toxic Micro-organisms" (M. Herzberg, ed.), pp. 287–291. U. S. Dept. of Interior, Washington, D. C.

Suyama, M., and Uno, Y. (1957–1958). *Nippon Suisangaku Kaishi* **23**, 438; cited from *Chem. Abstr.* **53**, 4590 (1959).

Taft, C. M. (1945). *Tex. Rep. Biol. Med.* **3**, 339.

Tahara, Y. (1910). *Biochem.* **30**, 255.

Takahashi, D., and Inoko, Y. (1892). *Mitt. Med. Fak. Tokio* **1**, 375.

Takata, M., Moore, J. W., Kao, C. Y., and Fuhrman, F. A. (1966). *J. Gen. Physiol.* **49**, 977.

Takayanagi, Y., Kitamura, T., and Satoh, T. (1953). *Soc. Publ. Health Hokkaido, 5th Meet.* (cited from Asano and Itoh, 1962).

Tani, I. (1945). "A Study of the Toxicity of Japanese Fugu" (in Japanese). Teikoku Tosho, Tokyo.

Taylor, J., and McCoy, J. H. (1969). *In* "Food-Borne Infections and Intoxications" (H. Reiman, ed.), pp. 3–72. Academic Press, New York.

Tsuda, K. (1966). *Naturwissenshaften* **53**, 171.

Tybring, O. (1886). *Bull. U. S. Fish Comm.* **6**, 148.

Van Wagtendonk, W. J., Fuhrman, F. A., Tatum, E. L., and Field, J. (1942). *Biol. Bull.* **83**, 137.

von Franque, A. (1858). *Deut. Klin.* **10**, 133.

Wakely, J. F., Fuhrman, G. J., Fuhrman, F. A., Fischer, H. G., and Mosher, H. S. (1966). *Toxicon* **3**, 195.

Walford, L. A. (1931). "Handbook of Common Commercial and Game Fishes of California," Fish Bull. No. 37. California Dept. of Fish and Game.

Waterfield, C. J., and Evans, M. H. (1972). *Experientia* **28**, 670.

Witthaus, R. A. (1911). "Manual of Toxicology," 2nd ed. Wm. Wood, New York.

Woodward, R. B. (1964). *Pure Appl. Chem.* **9**, 49.

Yokoo, A. (1950. *J. Chem. Soc. Jap. Pure Chem. Sect.* **71**, 590.

Yudkin, W. H. (1945). *J. Cell. Comp. Physiol.* **25**, 85.

Zlatogoroff, S. I., and Soloviev, M. N. (1927). *J. Amer. Med. Ass.* **88**, 2024.

4

□ □ □

SHELLFISH, FISH, AND ALGAE

Edward J. Schantz

I. Introduction

In many areas throughout the world man has been poisoned by eating certain fish. Many of these fish acquire the poison through the food chain from poisonous algae. Until recently, man has not considered seriously the direct consumption of algae as a source of food and, therefore, has not been confronted with the problem. However, domestic animals have been poisoned by the direct consumption of poisonous algae by drinking from lakes and ponds where heavy growth of the algae has taken place.

Hundreds of species of freshwater and marine organisms are known to be venomous or poisonous and most of these are described by Halstead (1962). However, only a few of them present serious food poisoning problems for man and his domestic animals. The important problems may be classed as (1) fish and shellfish that become poisonous as a result of consuming toxic or poisonous algae, such as many bivalves (mussels, clams, and oysters) and the ciguatoxic fishes; (2) fish that are intrinsically poisonous or produce the poison within their body, such as tetrodons or pufferfishes; and (3) poisonous algae that may get into drinking water and foods or feeds.

The purpose of this chapter is to describe the nature of these poisons, symptoms or signs of poisoning, and means of control or prevention. Reviews related to these subjects have been written by Halstead (1962), Dack (1957), Shilo (1967), Gorham (1960), Russell (1968), Schantz (1968, 1970), and Wills (1966).

II. Fish and Shellfish Poisons Produced by Algae

A. SHELLFISH POISONS

1. Paralytic Type of Poisons

Shellfish constitute one of the important seafoods for human consumption. In certain seacoast areas shellfish become extremely poisonous and cause paralysis and death in humans and animals. In most cases the shellfish do not produce the poison but acquire it from certain marine dinoflagellates that grow in the water where the shellfish feed. A classic example in this case is the relation of the toxic marine dinoflagellate, *Gonyaulax catenella,* to the sporadic occurrence of paralytic shellfish poisoning reported by Sommer and Meyer (1937), and Sommer *et al.* (1937) at the University of California. Prior to this time the cause of the sporadic occurrence of the poison in shellfish was unknown and very puzzling to persons who enjoyed shellfish, and to public health officials.

Shellfish that may have been safe to eat for generations, suddenly, and for no apparent reason, would become extremely poisonous. The shellfish would remain so for 1–3 weeks and then, for no apparent reason, become safe for human consumption again. During several outbreaks of shellfish poisoning along the central California coast between 1920 and 1937, the University of California investigators observed the presence of a particular microscopic dinoflagellate in the water around mussel beds where the mussels were poisonous. These workers identified this organism as *Gonyaulax catenella* and found that it contained a poison that produced symptoms in mice similar to those of extracts of poisonous mussels. Their work showed that the mussels acquired the poisonous properties through the food chain and that the mussels possess a mechanism in the dark gland or hepatopancreas that binds the poison and prevents it from causing any harm to the physiology of the mussel. This dark gland usually contains 95% or more of the poison found in a mussel. Mussels gradually destroy or excrete the bound poison so that within 1–3 weeks after the bloom of the dinoflagellate has subsided they are free of poison and safe for human consumption. However, in some clams, such as the Alaska butter clam, the poison apparently moves from the hepatopancreas to the siphon where it is bound and may be retained for many months before decreasing to a safe level (Schantz and Magnusson, 1964). The poison that is bound in the shellfish is readily released when consumed by man.

The regions of the world where paralytic shellfish poisoning has occurred most often are around the North Sea, the north Atlantic coast of America, the north Pacific coast of America from central California to the Aleutian Islands, the coastal areas of Japan, South Africa, and New Zealand. In general, these areas are 30° or more north or south latitude.

Several other species of dinoflagellates are poisonous. The main ones reported in recent years are *G. catenella*, which has been found along the Pacific coast of North America (Sommer and Meyer, 1937); *G. acatenella* along the coast of British Columbia (Prakash and Taylor, 1966), and *G. tamarensis* along the north Atlantic coast of North America and Europe (Needler, 1949; Prakash, 1963; Robinson, 1968). These organisms are listed in Table I. Whenever

TABLE I

Toxins Produced by Various Algae

Species	Common location	Biological characteristics	Chemical characteristics
Gonyaulax catenella	Pacific coast of North America	Toxic to all higher animals; predators bind toxin; poison blocks sodium influx in nerve cells	Among most potent poisons; low mol wt (372); water-soluble tetra-hydropurine
Gonyaulax acatenella	Pacific coast of North America	Similar to *G. catenella* poison	Not characterized
Gonyaulax tamarensis	Atlantic coast of North America	Appears similar to *G. catenella* poison	Appears similar to *G. catenella* poison
Gonyaulax polyedra[a]	California coast	Toxic to mice and fish; produces poison only under some conditions	Somewhat similar to *G. catenella* poison
Gonyaulax monilata	Gulf of Mexico	Toxic to fish	Not characterized
Pyrimidium phoenus	North Sea	Similar to *G. catenella* poison	Not characterized
Exuviaella mariae-lebouriae	Japan	Causes fatty degeneration of liver and kidney	Not characterized
Gymnodinium breve	Gulf of Mexico	Toxic to fish and mice; may be several poisons	One poison is lipid-soluble; mol wt 600–1500

Gymnodinium veneficum	Isolated from the English Channel	Toxic to fish and mice	High molecular weight; water-soluble
Cyanophyta; Blue-Green Algae			
Microcystis aeruginosa	Shallow freshwater lakes	Toxic to many animals (FDF)[b]	Cyclic polypeptide of 10 amino acid units; mol wt about 1200; water-soluble
Anabaena flos-aquae	Shallow freshwater lakes	Toxic to many animals; kills faster than M. aeruginosa (VFDF)[c]	Water-soluble
Schizothrix calcicola[e]	Pacific Ocean	Somewhat like ciguatera poisoning in man	Not characterized
Caulepra (several species)[c]	Western Pacific Ocean	Dizziness in man	Not characterized
Chrysophyta, Yellow-Brown Algae; Phytoflagellates			
Pyrmnesium parvum	Brackish water ponds and estuarine water	Toxic to fish and all gill-breathing animals; potent hemolytic agent	Water-soluble; non-dialyzable thermolabile; may be a saponin-like compound

[a]This species has been proposed as a food (see Patton et al., 1967).
[b]FDF, fast death factor (see Gorham, 1960).
[c]VFDF, very fast death factor (see Gorham, 1960).
[d]This species produces a poison but its relation to ciguatera poisoning from eating certain fish is speculative.
[c]Several species of Caulepra, when eaten by man, cause dizziness, but the symptoms are not well defined.

environmental conditions are right these organisms grow out and may persist for 1–3 weeks in a particular area. The amount of poison in the shellfish depends upon the number of poisonous organisms in the water and the amount of water filtered by the shellfish. Along the California coast mussels became too toxic for human consumption when 200 or more G. *catenella* cells were found per milliliter of water. This organism, like many other species of plankton, will produce a visible "red tide" when the count reaches 20,000 or more per milliliter.

Symptoms of shellfish poisoning may be apparent within 30 minutes after eating poisonous shellfish. The symptoms begin with a numbness in the lips and finger tips, followed by progressive paralysis and death from respiratory paralysis in 2–12 hours depending upon the magnitude of the dose. If a person survives 24 hours, the prognosis is good. Those who survive usually show no lasting effects from the ordeal. The dose to produce symptoms, derived from accidental cases of poisoning, may be only a few hundred mouse units and death may occur in humans from consuming 3000–5000 mouse units (Bond and Medcof, 1958). [A mouse unit (MU) is defined as the minimum amount to kill a 20-gm mouse in 15 minutes.] One small mussel weighing about 50 gm, that has consumed high concentrations of the poisonous organisms, may contain several lethal doses or as much as 20,000 to 30,000 MU. There is no known antidote for the poison. Because death appears to result from respiratory paralysis, artificial respiration has been used and believed successful, at least in borderline cases (Meyer, 1953).

The poison from poisonous California mussels and Alaska butter clams (called saxitoxin) was isolated in pure form in 1954 (Schantz *et al.*, 1957; Mold *et al.*, 1957). The purification of the poison from extracts of mussels and clams was accomplished by ion exchange chromatography on carboxylic acid resins, followed by chromatography on acid-washed alumina in absolute ethanol. By this technique a white hygroscopic product was obtained that had a potency of 5500 MU/mg solids. The purified poison is a dibasic salt pk_a at 8.2 and 11.5, is very soluble in water and quite stable to heat. Its molecular formula, as the hydrochloride salt, is $C_{10}H_{17}O_4N_7 \cdot 2HCl$ (molecular weight 372). It has no ultraviolet absorption, gives positive Benedict-Behre and Jaffe tests and is completely detoxified by mild catalytic reduction with the uptake of 1 mole of hydrogen per mole of poison at atmospheric pressure (Schantz *et al.*, 1957, 1961; Mold *et al.*, 1957).

The poison in shellfish must be detected with suitable animals. Because the poison does not affect the physiology and appearance of the shellfish there are no distinguishing characteristics between poisonous and nonpoisonous specimens to serve as a guide to a person collecting them. The only practical means of detecting the poison is by bioassay with mice, as originally devised by Sommer and Meyer (1937). The curve relating time of death to mouse units may be constructed from the following data. Death times of 3, 4, 5, 6, 7, 8, and 15 minutes are equivalent to 3.7, 2.5, 1.9, 1.6, 1.4, 1.3, and 1 MU, respectively. Although the mouse unit was originally defined in terms of the amount that will kill a 20-gm mouse in 15 minutes, the most consistent results are obtained when the death time is between 4 and 8 minutes (Schantz *et al.*, 1958). The weight of the mouse is a factor in the quantitative assay. Usually mice weighing between 19 and 21 gm are used where the variation due to weight is insignificant or about ± 3%.

The United States Food and Drug Administration has set standards of acceptance for the paralytic poison in shellfish to be not more than 400 MU, or about 80 $\mu g/100$ gm of shellfish meats. To put the assay on a standard basis the purified poison is used as a comparison. The procedure, including the use of the purified poison for comparison, has been made the official method of assay for paralytic shellfish poison by the Association of Official Agricultural Chemists (Schantz *et al.*, 1958; McFarren, 1959). Essentially the assay consists of heating a mixture of 100 gm of shellfish meats and 100 ml of water, adjusted to pH about 2, to boiling. Serial dilutions of the cooled clarified extract adjusted to pH about 4 are injected intraperitoneally into white mice weighing 19–21 gm. From the death times, as described above, the amount of poison in 100 gm of meats is calculated. In carrying out the assay, one or two mice are given 1 ml of the solution to obtain the approximate potency. In routine checking, three mice are used on a final dilution. To comply with the official method, 10 mice are used on the final dilution.

The best means of control of shellfish poisoning is direct sampling of the shellfish beds and assaying these for poison content. Many government agencies carry out assays periodically from May to October to check for the poison where shellfish are collected for food. If the shellfish become dangerously poisonous, warnings are posted and publicized. In spite of these warnings, however, some persons will collect shellfish for food because they are in the habit of doing so and the shellfish were perfectly good to eat from the preceding collection. Education of the public by Public Health agencies regarding the dangers of the sporadic occurrence of the poison and its cause is very important, especially in the areas where shellfish poisoning is common. This type of education no doubt is responsible for the reduced occurrences of poisoning in recent years. Regulations on the commercial collection and processing of shellfish are described by the U.S. Public Health Service (1959).

As mentioned previously, the poison in the Alaska butter clam and to some extent in other species, presents a somewhat complicated problem commercially in that the bulk of the poison in the clam is retained in the siphon for long periods of time. The butter clam is one of the most palatable of the species of clams and is an important food item in the economy of Alaska. Another difficulty in handling the problems of poison in clams and other shellfish is that the poison is quite stable to heating. Canned clams processed at 240°F in the normal manner may still contain 50% or more of the poison. Attempts to destroy the poison in clams by increasing the pH during processing were successful only when the pH was high enough to destroy the palatability of the clams. Removing the siphons, which contain 60–80% of the poison in the clams, will sometimes reduce the poison sufficiently to comply with the maximum limit of 400 MU/100 gm wet meats. Transplanting poisonous clams to beds where the clams are not poisonous required a year to show any appreciable decrease in the poison content.

These poisons are among the most potent known to man. In terms of purified poison, 1 MU, as defined previously, is equal to 0.18 μg. The intravenous dose for a rabbit weighing 1 kg is 3–4 μg. If it is assumed that 3000–5000 MU is a lethal dose for man, as indicated from accidental cases, then the weight of poison to cause death in man is 0.54–0.9 mg by oral dose. These poisons have become of special interest to physiologists because they block the propagation of impulses in nerves and skeletal muscle without depolarization. Evans (1964) and Kao and Nishiyama (1965) found that the block is due to some specific interference with the increase in sodium permeability, normally associated with excitation, and the passage of a nerve impulse. This action is specific for sodium and appears not to affect any other ions in the cell. The action is similar to that of tetrodotoxin from the puffer fish. (See Section III.)

2. Other Types of Shellfish Poisons

Other types of poisons have been found in shellfish after the consumption of dinoflagellates that have caused a variety of diseases in man after eating the shellfish (see Table I).

Nakazima (1968) has found that the poisonous properties of shellfish in Lake Hamana in Japan is due to the consumption of a poisonous dinoflagellate, *Exuviaella mariae-lebouriae.* The shellfish implicated in this case were oysters or asari and when consumed by man produce anorexia, abdominal pain, nausea, vomiting, constipation, and headache within the first few days, followed by hemorrhagic spots on the skin, bleeding from the mucous membranes and acute yellow atrophy of the liver. Several hundred cases have been reported in the area of Lake Hamana with more than 100 deaths. The toxic principle is found in the liver or dark gland of the bivalves and has been isolated by Japanese investigators. It is quite stable to heating and causes intoxication in many animals by both the oral and intraperitoneal route. Although the occurrence of this organism seems to have been limited to one particular area of Japan, the possibility of its occurrence in other areas of the world should not be overlooked by public health officials and persons in the shellfish industries. Detection of the poison is carried out by assay with mice.

In another case McFarren *et al.* (1965) have reported that oysters from the west coast of Florida, where they had been feeding on *Gymnidinium breve,* caused sickness in humans and animals with symptoms similar to ciguatera poisoning. This type of poisoning

will be described subsequently. Also, the Japanese investigators
(Konosu *et al.*, 1968) have found a poison in crabs that appears to
be identical to saxitoxin, the poison isolated from *G. catenella.*

B. CIGUATERA POISONING

Ciguatera poisoning is common throughout the Caribbean area
and much of the Pacific area, particularly in the torrid zones. Investigators at the University of Hawaii (Banner *et al.*, 1963) have carried
out a long series of studies on various marine animals that produce
ciguatera-like poisoning. Perhaps as many as 300 species of fishes
have been implicated in ciguatera poisoning within the Caribbean
area and the equatorial areas of the Pacific Ocean, but only 15
to 20 species are usually concerned, including snappers, barracudas,
surgeonfishes, jacks, groupers, sea basses, sharks, and eels. The
various species are listed by Russel (1968). The first symptoms
of the poisoning may be tingling of the lips, tongue, and throat,
followed by a numbness in these areas. In other cases, the initial
symptoms consist of nausea, vomiting, metallic taste, dryness of
the mouth, abdominal cramps, diarrhea, headache, prostration,
chills, fever, general muscular pain, and other symptoms. Weakness
may become progressively worse until the intoxicated person is
unable to walk. Mortality rates are not high in this type of poisoning,
but in severe cases, death may result from various complications,
mainly cardiovascular collapse. Banner and co-workers (1963) have
studied the toxin from red snappers, one of the highly toxic fish
usually caught south of the Hawaiian Islands, and compared this
toxin to that from the moray eel and shark livers from sharks
in this same area. While the toxins from the various sources appear
to produce somewhat similar symptoms, there is evidence that the
toxin from each source is a mixture of toxic substances. This fact
has complicated investigations on the nature of the poisons causing
ciguatera. With comparatively few exceptions, the fishes responsible
for ciguatera poisoning are not uniformly and consistently
poisonous. Most poisonous fishes seem to be taken near shores,
rather than from deep waters. Furthermore, toxicity is not species-
specific. For these reasons it is believed that the poison causing

ciguatera originates in some of the marine algae and gets to the fish through the food chain. Cooper (1964) has reported the appearance of toxic fish with the sudden appearance of an alga that paralleled the reported distribution of toxic fish. The alga was identified as *Schizothrix calcicola*. Both water and lipid extracts of the alga contained toxins which produce symptoms in mice and mongoose similar to those of the extracts of fish. It is difficult to postulate how many different toxins have been encountered in the study on ciguatera. The appearance of many compounds in the chemical isolation may be due to degradation during treatment or some change in structure as it is consumed by different species of fish. Poisons have been isolated and characterized (Hessel, 1961; Banner *et al.*, 1963; Scheuer *et al.*, 1967). The poisons are stable to heat used in ordinary cooking and can be dried without loss of potency. They are quite soluble in lipid solvents, but soluble to some extent in water. There is no estimate of the dose required to cause sickness in humans but the purified preparations have been found lethal to mice (weight about 20 gm) at levels of about 25 μg down to 4 μg.

Due to the sporadic occurrence of ciguatera poisons, control for public safety is difficult. Medical and public health officials must be continually on the watch for cases that might indicate that fish in a certain area are becoming poisonous. Several species of algae in the Pacific area have been found to be poisonous, but their relationship to poisonous fish has not been established.

III. Poisonous Fish

A. PUFFERFISH POISON (PARALYTIC POISON)

Pufferfish poisoning has always been a problem in Japan. The pufferfish are sometimes referred to as blowfish, globefish, or fugufish. The toxic ones are included in the family *Tetraodontidae,* but not all the fish in this family possess the toxin. These are listed by Wills (1966). However, the choice edible species harbor the toxin, which is located in the liver, ovaries, and eggs (see chapter 3) of the female, and liver and testes of the male. Symptoms of pufferfish poisoning usually begin with a tingling or prickling sensation of the fingers and toes, lips, and tongue within a few minutes after eating poisonous fish. Nausea, vomiting, diarrhea, and epigastric pain may appear in some cases. As the intoxication deepens, the pupillary and corneal reflexes are lost and respiratory distress increases. If the dose is sufficient, death results from respiratory paralysis much like that of shellfish poisoning. The mortality rate of pufferfish poisoning is very high. The poison (tetrodotoxin) has been isolated from the ovaries and testes of the pufferfish in a highly purified form by Japanese and American workers and its chemical structure is known (Tsuda *et al.*, 1964; Woodward, 1964). See Chapter 3. It has a molecular weight of 329. It is much less soluble in water than saxitoxin and has an entirely different chemical structure, an aminoperhydroquinazoline compound compared to a substituted tetrahydropurine. One remarkable thing about tetrodotoxin and saxitoxin is that they both have an identical physiological action in that they block the diffusion of sodium ions into a nerve or muscle cell to inhibit the passage of an impulse. The potency of the two poisons in mice and other experimental animals is very similar. The dose for a mouse being about 0.2 μg and for a rabbit (1 kg) about 3–4 μg. It is assumed that the amount to cause death in humans is equivalent to the amount of saxitoxin to produce death in humans. Tetrodotoxin is identical in chemical structure to the poison from some species of salamanders, such as *Taricha torosa* found in California (Buchwald *et al.*, 1964).

Legislative control, aimed at preventing pufferfish poisoning in Japan, has undergone several forms, from outright prohibition of sale, to more realistic measures. These laws generally take the form of licensing handlers of tetrodon fish in special restaurants. License is granted if the individual is judged knowledgeable on the species and seasonal variations in toxicity, and capable of eviscerating toxic species of fish without cutting the liver and roe. The effectiveness of these measures can be appreciated from the fact that in well-managed restaurants, where considerable amounts of pufferfish are consumed, there is very seldom a case of poisoning, whereas puffers prepared and sold by persons not trained and licensed results in several hundred cases each year, with many deaths.

The heat stability of tetrodotoxin or pufferfish poison has been studied by Halstead and Bunker (1953) who found that after the usual commercial canning procedure, some of the toxicity that came in cut whole fish was lost, but not sufficiently for safe human consumption. Procedures included heating to 100°C for 10 minutes and heating under pressure at 116°C, but these steps did not inactivate the poison completely and one cannot rely upon processing alone to destroy the poison in canned fish. Assays for control measures on the poison are carried out with mice, using a procedure similar to that for shellfish poisons.

B. OTHER FISH POISONS

Poisoning from eating several other types of marine animals has caused sickness and in some cases death. These types are listed by Wills (1966), Dack (1957), and Halstead (1962), and include certain herring-like fishes of the Pacific (clupeoid poisoning), some of the snake mackerels (gempylid poisoning), sharks and dogfishes (elasmobranch poisoning), lampreys and hagfishes (cyclostome poisoning), squid and octopus (cephalopod poisoning), certain porpoises in the Yangtze and certain turtles. The common symptoms of poisoning in humans are nausea, vomiting, diarrhea, dyspnea, cyanosis, coma, and convulsions. The source of the poison in these marine organisms is not known, but until more information is forthcoming, it is assumed that the poison is produced by the animal and characteristic of a particular species.

IV. Poisonous Algae

A. DINOFLAGELLATES

The dinoflagellates are an important group of microorganisms that inhabit both fresh and marine waters. They possess attributes of both plant and animal life and have been described as algae,

protozoa, and protista. Most of them are able to manufacture their
own food by photosynthesis, but many require additional pre-
formed organic substances for growth and reproduction. The
known dinoflagellates that produce poison are mainly those of
marine origin (Schantz, 1971). These are listed in the first part
of Table I. As stated above the dinoflagellates, *Gonyaulax catenella,
Gonyaulax acatenella, Gonyaulax tamarensis, Pyrimidium phoenus,
Exuviaella mariae-lebouriae,* and *Gymnodinium breve* have been directly
involved in causing shellfish to become poisonous, resulting in food
poisoning in humans.

Some other dinoflagellates are poisonous, but not all have been
known to cause shellfish poisoning. Schradie and Bliss (1962)
reported that *Gonyaulax polyedra,* which occurs along the southern
coast of California, is poisonous but it never has been proven to
cause any type of shellfish poisoning. Because of the prolific growth
of this organism in cultures it has been proposed as a means of
producing feed for cattle (Patton *et al.,* 1967). *Gonyaulax monilata,*
a dinoflagellate common in the Gulf of Mexico, produces a poison
that is toxic to fish. Ray and Aldrich (1965), have found that
Gonyaulax monilata is not toxic to chicks and, as far as is known,
is not toxic to mice and other warm-blooded animals. Oysters in
the Gulf of Mexico do not filter water when exposed to *G. monilata.*
Abbott and Ballantine (1957), found that *Gymnidinium veneficum,*
isolated from the English Channel, produces a poison that is toxic
to both fish and mice but has not been known to cause shellfish
poisoning. Ray and Aldrich (1967), Spikes *et al.* (1968), and Martin
and Chatterjee (1969), found that the dinoflagellate *Gymnidinium
breve* produces a poison extractable in lipid solvents that is toxic
to fish, chicks, and mice. Recently these investigators purified some
poisons from this organism and characterized them to some extent.
One appears to be a neurotoxin and causes death in animals by
respiratory failure. It has a potency of about 100 LD/mg for mice.
There may be many other dinoflagellates throughout the world
that produce poisons, but we are lacking information on these
organisms in respect to the poisonous substances that they may
produce. As mentioned before, such discoveries usually have been
made when food poisoning has occurred in man or animals in

some way that is related to a certain dinoflagellate or other organism.

The only poison from the dinoflagellates that has been characterized to a great extent is that from *Gonyaulax catenella,* the predominant poisonous dinoflagellate along the Pacific coast. This organism has been grown in axenic culture and the poison obtained in pure form by a procedure similar to that used for the purification of the poison from clams and mussels. The chemical structure of this poison is identical to saxitoxin, the poison obtained from poisonous California mussels and Alaska butter clams (Schantz *et al.,* 1966). This fact indicates that the poison is bound in the dark gland of mussels and siphon of clams without a change in its chemical structure. The poison produced by *G. tamarensis* in axenic culture has also been isolated in pure form. Its chemical structure is somewhat different than that of the poison from *G. catenella* (Schantz, 1971), but the physiological action of the two poisons is identical.

B. BLUE-GREEN ALGAE

Several species of the blue-green algae have caused public health problems and heavy economic loss by killing domestic animals. *Anabaena flos-aquae* and *Microcystis aeruginosa* have produced blooms in shallow freshwater lakes throughout the world, and have killed thousands of cattle, horses, sheep, hogs, certain fowl, and dogs that drank water containing large numbers of these organisms. Concentrations usually become high on the leeward side of freshwater lakes after heavy algal growths in shallow waters. Such occurrences have been reported in North America, particularly from North and South Dakota, Minnesota, Iowa, Wisconsin, Illinois, and Michigan in United States and from the provinces of Alberta, Saskatchewan, Manitoba, and Ontario in Canada (Grant and Hughes, 1953). The occurrence of blooms of toxic algae in these areas have been studied by several investigators in the United States and Canada and recently reviewed by Gorham (1960). Similar blooms of toxic algae have been reported in Russia, Brazil, Australia, and South Africa (Gorham, 1960).

Of the several poisons and toxins that have been identified in blue-green algal cultures, only two have been isolated in pure form and characterized chemically and physically. The first of these was the so-called "fast death factor" (FDF) found in certain unialgal cultures of the blue-green alga *M. aeruginosa* reported by Bishop *et al.* (1959) of the National Research Council, Canada, in 1959. These workers termed the toxin the "fast death factor" because a minimum lethal dose by intraperitoneal injection killed mice in 30–60 minutes in contrast to another toxin found in these preparations that caused death in 4–48 hours. This they called the "slow death factor" (SDF). After considerable effort in selecting strains, a unialgal culture of *M. aeruginosa,* designated NRC-1, was obtained that produced the FDF and SDF in quantities equal to those of the natural state but with the advantages of having control of the critical factors for toxin production. Thus these investigators were able to produce a continuous laboratory bloom on a scale sufficient to yield 1–2 kg of freeze-dried cells per month. The medium was composed of demineralized water with 0.04% $NaNO_3$ as a nitrogen source plus various inorganic salts and citrate as described by Hughes *et al.* (1958). Cultures were illuminated and held at 25°C for 4 days for maximum toxin production. The algal cells were agglomerated with a small amount of aluminum sulfate and HCl to permit rapid centrifugation. Fresh cells were not toxic to mice but became toxic when they were frozen and thawed, sonic-disintegrated, or decomposed by semianaerobic incubation. The toxin (FDF) was extracted from the decomposed algal cells with water and subjected to electrophoresis on paper, first under acidic conditions and then under alkaline conditions, yielding a highly purified toxic component that killed mice at a minimum lethal dose of about 9 μg in a 20-gm mouse, or 450 μg/kg. It is a moderately toxic substance. Its specific toxicity, in terms of minimum lethal mouse doses per gram of solids, is 1.1×10^5. Because the FDF formed only on the decomposition of the algal cells, it is believed to be an endotoxin. It was found to be a cyclic polypeptide made up of 10 amino acid units as follows: 1 residue each of L-aspartic acid, D-serine, L-valine, and L-ornithine and 2 residues each of L-glutamic acid, L-alanine, and L-leucine. The molecular weight is about 1200. The occurrence of the unnatural amino acid D-serine in the peptide is interesting. The toxin did not react with reagents for terminal amino acids of proteins, so it was assumed that the peptide must be cyclic. The amino acid sequence and structure have not yet been determined.

The "slow death factor" associated with the algal cultures is believed to result from the decomposition of the bacteria in the culture, and its presence could be demonstrated by differential centrifugation of the algae from the bacteria and allowing decomposition to take place. The decomposed algal cells yielded the FDF; the bacterial cells yielded the SDF.

The poison produced by *Anabaena flos-aquae* acts even more rapidly than the FDF and was termed by the Canadian workers the "very fast death factor" (VFDF). However, this toxin has been obtained only from natural cultures and has not been isolated or characterized. It is water soluble and probably lower in molecular weight than the FDF (Gorham, 1960).

The toxin of the blue-green freshwater alga, *M. aeruginosa* (FDF), studied by the Canadians (Bishop *et al.*, 1959; Gorham, 1960), is toxic to a great variety of animals except waterfowl, indicating that the waterfowl have a mechanism to protect them against the toxin. In most animals, the FDF produces pallor followed by violent convulsions, prostration, and death. Upon autopsy, the liver has a mottled appearance caused by cellular breakdown. On the other hand, the toxin from *Anabaena flos-aquae* (VFDF) will kill waterfowl (Gorham, 1960). As mentioned previously, the latter toxin kills mice very rapidly, with death preceded by paralysis, tremors, and mild convulsions. Upon autopsy, the liver appears normal. It is apparent, therefore, that these two toxins must be different in their chemical structure. The FDF has no antigenic activity and no antibiotic activity, although its structure as a cyclic polypeptide would suggest this possibility.

Jackim and Gentile (1968) have isolated and purified a poison from the blue-green alga, *Aphanizomenon flos-aquae,* that is chemically similar to the poison from the dinoflagellate *G. catenella* (saxitoxin). The physiological action of this poison is similar to that of the poison from *G. catenella* (Sawyer *et al.,* 1968). Recently certain species of *Caulepra,* a marine blue-green alga, have been found to contain toxic substances (M. S. Doty, and G. Aguilar-Santos, personal communication).

C. YELLOW-BROWN ALGAE

Another toxin of great interest is one produced by one of the yellow-brown alga, *Pyrmnesium parvum.* This alga grows in the brackish water ponds and estuary waters and produces a toxin that is lethal to fish and all gill-breathing animals. The toxin produced by the organism inhibits the transfer of oxygen across the gill membranes and has been a great problem in the commercial carp tanks in Israel. Several investigators in Israel have isolated and studied the toxin to a great extent (Otterstrom and Steemann-Nielsen, 1939; Reich *et al.,* 1965; Parnas, 1963; Shilo and Rosenberger, 1960). It is nondialyzable, thermolabile, and believed to be a saponin-like compound that is a potent hemolytic agent. The toxin probably exceeds 100,000 in molecular weight.

References

Abbott, B. C., and Ballantine, D. (1957). *J. Mar. Biol. Ass. U. K.* **36,** 169.

Banner, A. H., Helfrich, P., Scheuer, P. J., and Yoshida, T. (1963). *Proc. Gulf Carib. Fish Inst., 16th Annu. Sess.* p. 48.

Bishop, C. T., Amet, E.F.L.J., and Gorham, P.R. (1959). *Can. J. Biochem. Physiol.* **37,** 453.

Bond, R. M., and Medcof, J. C. (1958). *Can. Med. Ass. J.* **79,** 19.

Buchwald, H. D., Durham, L., Fischer, H. G., Harada, R., Mosher, H. S., Kao, C. Y., and Fuhrman, F. A. (1964). *Science* **140,** 295.

Cooper, M. J. (1964). *Pac. Sci.* **18,** 411.

Dack, G. M. (1957). "Food Poisoning." Univ. of Chicago Press, Chicago, Illinois.

Evans, M. H. (1964). *Brit. J. Pharmacol. Chemother.* **22,** 478.

Gorham, P. R. (1960). *Can. Vet. J.* **1,** 235.

Grant, G. A., and Hughes, E. O. (1953). *Can. J. Pub. Health* **44,** 334.

Halstead, B. W. (1962). "Poisonous and Venomous Marine Animals," Vol. 1. US Govt. Printing Office, Washington, D.C.

Halstead, B. W., and Bunker, N. C. (1953). *Calif. Fish Game* **39,** 219.

Hessel, D. W. (1961). *Toxicol. Appl. Pharmacol.* **3,** 574.

Hessel, D. W., Halstead, B. W., and Peckham, N. H. (1960). *Ann. N.Y. Acad. Sci.* **90,** 788.

Hughes, E. O., Gorham, P. R., and Zehnder, A. (1958). *Can. J. Microbiol.* **4,** 225.

Jackim, E., and Gentile, J. (1968). *Science* **162,** 915.

Kao, C. Y., and Nishiyama, A. (1965). *J. Physiol. (London)* **180,** 50.

Konosu, S., Inone, A., Noguchi, T., and Hashimoto, Y. (1968). *Toxicon* **6,** 113.

McFarren, E.F. (1959). *J. Ass. Offic. Agr. Chem.* **42,** 263.

McFarren, E. F., Tanabe, H., Silva, F. J., Wilson, W. B., Campbell, J. E., and Lewis, K. H. (1965). *Toxicon* **3,** 111.

Martin, D. F., and Chatterjee, A. B. (1969). *Nature (London)* **221,** 59.

Meyer, K. F. (1953). *N. Engl. J. Med.* **249,** 848.

Mold, J. D., Bowden, J. P., Stanger, D. W., Maurer, J. E., Lynch, J. M., Wyler, R. S., Schantz, E. J., and Riegel, B. (1957). *J. Amer. Chem. Soc.* **79,** 5235.

Nakazima, M. (1968). *Bull. Jap. Soc. Sci. Fish.* **34,** 130.

Needler, A. B. (1949). *J. Fish. Res. Bd. Can.* **7,** 490.

Otterstrøm, C. V., and Steemann-Nielsen, E. (1939). *Rep. Dan. Biol. Sta.* **44,** 5.

Parnas, I. (1963). *Isr. J. Zool.* **12,** 15.

Patton, S., Chandler, P. T., Kalan, E. B., Loeblich, A. R., III, Fuller, G., and Benson, A. A. (1967). *Science* **158,** 789.

Prakash, A. (1963). *J. Fish, Res. Bd. Can.* **20,** 983.

Prakash, A., and Taylor, F. J. R. (1966). *J. Fish. Res. Bd. Can.* **23,** 1265.

Ray, S. M., and Aldrich, D. V. (1965). *Science* **148,** 1748.

Ray, S. M., and Aldrich, D. V. (1967). *In* "Animal Toxins" (F. E. Russel and P. R. Sanders, eds.), pp. 75–83. Permagon, Oxford.

Reich, K., Bergmann, F., and Kidron, M. (1965). *Toxicon* **3,** 33.

Robinson, G. A. (1968). *Nature (London)* **220,** 22.

Russell, F. E. (1968). *In* "Safety of Foods" (H. D. Graham, ed.), p. 68. Avi, Westport, Connecticut.

Sawyer, P. J., Gentile, J. H., and Sasner, J. J. (1968). *Can. J. Microbiol.* **14,** 1199.

Schantz, E. J. (1968). *In* "Biochemistry of Some Foodborne Microbial Toxins" (R. I. Mateles and G. N. Wogan, eds.), p. 51. MIT Press, Cambridge, Massachusetts.

Schantz, E. J. (1970). *In* "Properties and Products of Algae." Plenum, New York.

Schantz, E. J. (1971). *In* "Microbial Toxins" Vol. VII, (S. Kadis, A. Ciegler, and S. J. Ajl, eds.), pp. 3–26. Academic Press, New York.

Schantz, E. J., and Magnusson, H. W. (1964). *J. Protozool.* **11,** 239.

Schantz, E. J., Mold, J. D., Stanger, D. W., Shavel, J., Riel, F. J., Bowden, J. P., Lynch, J. M., Wyler, R. W., Riegel, B., and Sommer, H. (1957). *J. Amer. Chem. Soc.* **79,** 5230.

Schantz, E. J., McFarren, E. F., Schafer, E. L., and Lewis, K. H. (1958). *J. Ass. Offic. Agr. Chem.* **41,** 160.

Schantz, E. J., Mold, J. D., Howard, W. L., Bowden, J. P., Stanger, D. W., Lynch, J. M., Wintersteiner, O. P., Dutcher, J. D., Walters, D. R., and Riegel, B. (1961). *Can. J. Chem.* **39,** 2117.

Schantz, E. J., Lynch, J. M., Vayvada, G., Matsumoto, K., and Rapoport, H. (1966). *Biochemistry* **5,** 1191.

Scheuer, P. J., Takahashi, W., Tsutsumi, J., and Yoshido, T. (1967). *Science* **155,** 1268.

Schradie, J., and Bliss, C. A. (1962). *Lloydia* **25,** 214.

Shilo, M. (1967). *Bacteriol. Rev.* **31,** 180.

Shilo, M., and Rosenberger, R. F. (1960). *Ann. N.Y. Acad. Sci.* **90,** 866.

Sommer, H., and Meyer, K. F. (1937). *Arch. Pathol.* **24,** 560.

Sommer, H., Whedon, W. F., Kofoid, C. A., and Stohler, R. (1937). *Arch. Pathol.* **24,** 537.

Spikes, J. J., Ray, S. M., Aldrich, D. V., and Nash, J. B. (1968). *Toxicon* **5,** 171.

Tsuda, K., Tachikawa, R., Sakai, K., Tamura, C., Amahasu, O., Kawamura, M., and Ikuma, S. (1964). *Chem. Pharm. Bull.* **12,** 642.

U. S. Public Health Service. (1959). "Manual of Recommended Practice for Sanitary Control of the Shellfish Industry," Part I. U.S. Pub. Health Serv., Washington, D.C.

Wills, J. H., Jr. (1966). *Acad. Sci. – Nat. Res. Counc., Publ.* **1354,** 147.

Woodward, R. B. (1964). *Pure Appl. Chem.* **9,** 49.

5

□ □ □

NITROSAMINES

N. P. Sen

131

I. Introduction

With the advent of modern technology and the availability of sophisticated analytical techniques the problem of toxic compounds in foods, both naturally occurring and artificially added, has received increasing attention due to concern over public health. The occurrences of goitrogens, antivitamins, cycasin, pesticides, mycotoxins, seafood toxins, and toxic minerals in various foods are a few examples. The presence of nitrosamines in foods is one of the problems that has aroused a great deal of controversy in recent years. Nitrates and nitrites, which are used as food additives, have been indicated as major factors responsible for aggravating the problem. The episode began in early times when it was accidently noticed that meat preserved with rock salt developed some red patches after cooking. It was later discovered that metallic nitrates, present as impurities in the rock salt, were responsible for this phenomenon. Subsequent observations led to the discovery that it was the nitrite, which was produced from nitrate by the action of microorganisms present in the meat, that reacted with the meat pigments to form the stable red color. In recent years nitrates and nitrites have been deliberately used to produce uniform red color in preserved meats and this practice led to the development of the modern curing process. Although nitrates and nitrites were chiefly used for producing the red color in meats, these compounds were also found to have some preservative action against

Clostridia. Later, nitrates and nitrites became acceptable as preservatives in other foods such as fish and cheese.

Nitrates and nitrites are physiologically active in man and animals and many of the clinical effects such as vasodilatation, lowering of blood pressure, and methemoglobin formation are well known. Some of these aspects will be discussed later in the text. However, the situation has become more complicated by the recent findings that nitrite and secondary or tertiary amines in foods may combine to form nitrosamines which are potent carcinogens. Magee and Barnes (1956) first reported the carcinogenicity of dimethylnitrosamine (DMN) in rats and subsequent reports (Schmaehl and Preussmann, 1959; Druckrey *et al.,* 1967) established that DMN as well as many other *N*-nitrosamines are carcinogenic to a wide range of species causing cancer at different sites of the body. Some can cause cancer after only one dose, and some are powerful mutagens.

Although the initial research work on the toxicity and carcinogenicity of nitrosamines was stimulated by indications of human toxicity arising from industrial usage it was not until 1960 that the possible occurrence of these compounds in our environment, other than contamination from industrial sources, was suspected. The first evidence that nitrosamines could be present in food was provided by Norwegian workers who were investigating a liver disease in fur-bearing animals (Bøhler, 1960, 1962). A similar hepatic disorder was later observed in cattle and sheep (Koppang, 1964). Extensive studies by Koppang and his associates (Koppang, 1964; Koppang and Helgebostad, 1966) revealed that the toxic effect was associated with feeding of herring meal that had been preserved with sodium nitrite. The responsible factor was subsequently isolated from the meal and identified as DMN (Ender *et al.,* 1964). It was also established that DMN in the toxic meal originated from the interactions of sodium nitrite and various methylamines, mainly dimethylamine and trimethylamine, naturally occurring in the fish.

These findings aroused a great deal of concern among scientists and health officials because of the possibility of occurrences of nitrosamines in human foods. The clear indications, that if enough DMN could be formed in fish meal to show an acute toxic effect and sometimes prove fatal to animals, suggested the possibility of the presence of smaller amounts of DMN or other nitrosamines in human foods, especially those rich in amines and nitrite. Added to this was the concern that nitrite may react with dietary supplies of secondary and tertiary amines in the acidic environment of the human stomach to form nitrosamines (Sander, 1967a; Sen *et al.,* 1969b). Clearly, then, the possibility of the occurrence of nitrosamines in foods or their potential formation from precursors in the human stomach are matters of real concern.

Nitrates, nitrites, and amines all play a key role in the formation of nitrosamines. A knowledge of the occurrence, formation, and interactions of these chemicals in foods is essential for full understanding of the problem. Since specific, sensitive, and accurate methods are necessary for obtaining meaningful results, precise analytical methodology is essential. A consideration of these areas will be made in greater detail. A recently published book (a companion volume of this monograph) entitled "Toxic Constituents of Plant Foodstuffs" (Liener, 1969) does not cover the occurrence of nitrosamines. Hence, it is appropriate to discuss briefly the subject of nitrosamines in foods of plant origin. Such a massive amount of work has been published on the biological actions of nitrosamines and other nitroso compounds that it is not possible to cover them all within the scope of this chapter. Therefore, an attempt will be made to summarize the important findings only, and discuss the implications with regard to the possible effect on human health.

II. Chemistry

A. STRUCTURE

The general formula of N-nitrosamines (or simply "nitrosamines") can be described as follows:

$$\begin{matrix} R_1 \\ \quad \diagdown \\ \qquad \qquad N{-}N{=}O \\ \quad \diagup \\ R_2 \end{matrix}$$

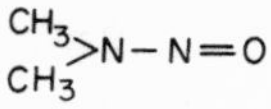

(I)

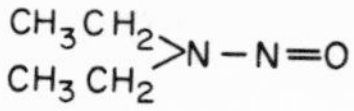

(II)

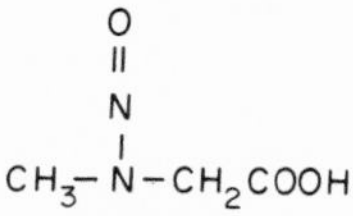

(III)

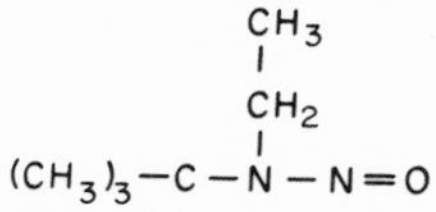

(IV)

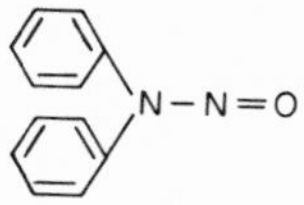

(V)

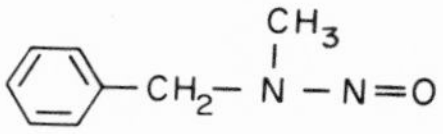

(VI)

(VII)

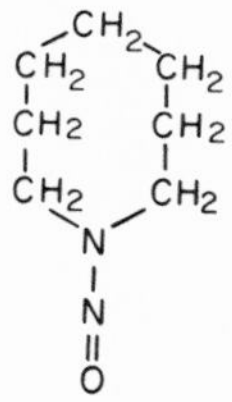

(VIII)

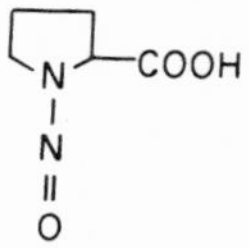

(IX)

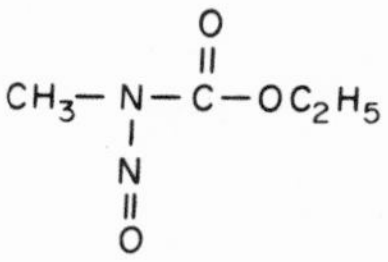

(X)

Fig. 1. Structural formulas of some typical nitroso compounds: (I) dimethylnitrosamine, (II) diethylnitrosamine, (III) nitrososarcosine, (IV) ethyl-*tert*-butylnitrosamine, (V) diphenylnitrosamine, (VI) methylbenzylnitrosamine, (VII) nitrosopyrrolidine, (VIII) nitrosoheptamethyleneimine, (IX) nitrosoproline, and (X) nitrosomethylurethane.

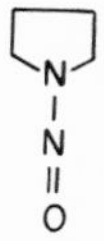

R₁ and R₂ can be either alkyl or aryl groups or, in some cases, alicyclic. For certain cyclic nitrosamines R₁ and R₂ may be replaced by a cyclic ring as in the case of nitrosopyrrolidine and nitrosoheptamethyleneimine (Fig. 1). Besides the nitrosamines there are many other carcinogenic N-nitroso compounds which could be present or formed in foods. These include nitrososarcosine, a nitroso amino acid, nitrosomethylurethane, and many others. The structural formulas of several common nitroso compounds are presented in Fig. 1. Note that the basic structure of all the compounds is similar and only the substituent groups (R₁ and R₂) have been changed. Due to their simplicity in structure and easy availability DMN and diethylnitrosamine (DEN) have found favor with scientists and have been widely used for various studies.

B. GENERAL PROPERTIES

The physical properties of nitrosamines vary widely depending on the nature and size of the substituent groups. This can be exemplified by the fact that DMN is an oily yellow liquid, bp 154°C, and it is miscible with water, ethanol, ether, or chloroform but only slightly soluble in nonpolar solvents such as *n*-pentane. Diphenylnitrosamine, on the other hand, is a yellow solid, mp 65°C, and only slightly soluble in ethanol and practically insoluble in water. It is, however, easily soluble in hot ethanol and chloroform. Di-*n*-octylnitrosamine is another extreme example. It is practically insoluble in polar solvents and highly lipophilic. The distribution coefficient (concentration in acetonitrile/concentration in heptane) of di-*n*-octylnitrosamine in acetonitrile-*n*-heptane is only 0.5 and that for DMN and methyl-2-hydroxyethylnitrosamine are 17.3 and 32.0, respectively (Eisenbrand *et al.,* 1969). Detailed physical properties such as solubility, melting and boiling points, density, ultraviolet absorptivity, refractive index, etc. of various nitrosamines have been published (Druckrey *et al.,* 1967; CRC Handbook of Chemistry and Physics, 1966–67; Fieser and Fieser, 1968). Various properties of several nitroso amino acids and cyclic nitrosamines have been reported by Lijinsky *et al.* (1969, 1970). Most of the dialkyl- and some of the alkylarylnitrosamines are steam-volatile and this property has been used for the separation of these compounds (Walters *et al.*, 1970; Eisenbrand *et al.*, 1970a). As nitrosamines are amides of nitrous acid they are nonbasic and insoluble in dilute acids (Noller, 1957).

C. SYNTHETIC PREPARATION

The nitrosamines are easily prepared by the action of nitrous acid on the corresponding secondary amines. For example, DMN is prepared by heating a mixture of equimolar quantities of dimethylamine hydrochloride and sodium nitrite in dilute hydrochloric acid. It is finally isolated in 80–90% yield as a yellow oil after distillation, extraction into ether, and further distillation through a fractionating column (Hatt, 1943). Nitrosomethylaniline can be similarly prepared from N-methylaniline in 93% yield (Hartman and Roll, 1943). Other nitrosating agents such as amylnitrite, nitrosyl chloride, or nitrosonium tetrafluoroborate have also been used to prepare nitrosamines in good yields (Fieser and Fieser, 1967). These reagents are particularly suitable for nitrosating amines which are insoluble in aqueous solution. Secondary aromatic amines produce nitrosamines just as do their aliphatic counterparts; both the diaryl and alkylaryl secondary amines easily form nitrosamines after treatment with nitrous acid or other nitrosating agents.

D. REACTIONS

The nitrosamines are highly photosensitive and easily decomposed by exposure to ultraviolet light, especially in the presence of strong acids. The mechanism of breakdown is complex but the main products of the decomposition are hyponitrous acid and secondary amines. Chow (1967) has studied the photochemistry of several nitroso compounds and concluded that the primary products are [NOH] and the corresponding alkylidineimines which subsequently hydrolyze to carbonyl compounds and secondary amines. Nitrosamines are stable to strong alkali and dilute acids but decompose to the original components on boiling with strong concentrated acids (Fieser and Fieser, 1968). The alkylnitrosamides are extremely unstable at alkaline pH and break down to diazoalkanes. In fact, nitrosomethylurethane is used in the laboratory for preparing diazomethane. Many of the nitrosamides decompose readily at neutral pH. The half-life of nitrosomethylurea, for example, is 125 hours at pH 4, 1.2 hours at pH 7, and only 0.1 hour at pH 8 (Druckrey *et al.*, 1967). Nitrosamines react vigorously with sodium azide and dilute hydrochloric acid with the formation of secondary amines and liberation of nitrogen and nitrous oxide. This reaction is used to distinguish the *C*-nitroso from the *C*-nitroso compounds which do not react with hydrazoic acid (Fiegl, 1955).

Nitrosamines can be reduced to the corresponding unsymmetrical hydrazines by treatment with suitable reducing agents. A mixture of zinc or tin and an acid, lithium aluminum hydride or sodium amalgam, can be used as the reducing agent. For example, DMN on treatment with zinc dust and acetic acid or lithium aluminum hydride produces *N,N*-dimethylhydrazine (Hatt, 1943; Serfontein and Hurter, 1966). On treatment with a more powerful reagent such as zinc and a mineral acid, methylphenylnitrosamine undergoes fission at the N—N linkage and produces methylphenylamine and ammonia (Fieser and Fieser, 1968). Aromatic *N*-nitrosamines readily undergo the well-known Fisher-Hepp rearrangement under the catalytic influence of hydrochloric acid. Thus, when a solution of *N*-nitroso-*N*-methylaniline (or methylphenylnitrosamine) in alcohol is mixed with concentrated hydrochloric acid and allowed to stand at room temperature, the compound rearranges to *p*-nitroso-*N*-methylaniline (Fieser and Fieser, 1968).

Nitrosamines are oxidized to nitramines by strong oxidizing agents such as pertrifluoroacetic acid, which is usually prepared *in situ* from hydrogen peroxide and trifluoroacetic acid or trifluoroacetic anhydride. Using the principle of this reaction a sensitive method for determining nitrosamines has been developed (Section V,C). The use of anhydrous pertrifluoroacetic acid, formed by mixing 90% hydrogen peroxide and an appropriate amount of trifluoroacetic anhydride, results in nearly 91% conversion of DEN to diethylnitramine (Emmons, 1954). Recently, Tolstikov and his associates (1971) have shown that *tert*-amyl hydroperoxide can effectively oxidize nitrosamines in the presence of MoCl₅ as a catalyst. Using this technique, these workers prepared dimethylnitramine (mp 54–55°C), nitromorpholine (mp 52–53°C) and nitropiperidine (mp −6°C) from the corresponding nitrosamines in 80% yields. Methyl nitrosourethane reacts with cysteine and glutathione at neutral pH. The reaction occurs at room temperature with evolution of gaseous nitrogen (Schoental, 1961, 1966). The main products are S-methylcysteine and S-ethoxycarbonylcystine. DMN and other dialkylnitrosamines are not known to react with sulfhydryl compounds at neutral pH.

III. Role of Nitrates, Nitrites, and Various Amino Compounds in the Formation of Nitrosamines in Foods

A. NITRATES AND NITRITES

Nitrates and nitrites occur widely in plants, water supplies, and soil. The natural level of these chemicals in animal tissues is, however, negligible (Stieglitz and Palmer, 1934). With increasing use of nitrogen fertilizers the levels of nitrate in vegetables have been shown to increase but with little or no effect on accumulation of nitrite (Lee et al., 1971). Extensive investigations have been carried out by various workers to determine the amounts of nitrate and nitrite in vegetable products and considerable amounts of data are available (Richardson, 1907; Wilson, 1943; Kilgore et al., 1963; Kamm et al., 1965). In general, common vegetables such as cabbage, cauliflower, beets, broccoli, celery, lettuce, parsley, radish, spinach, and turnips usually contain large amounts of nitrate but only traces of nitrite. However, under storage conditions nitrate in vegetables can be reduced to nitrite, as has been observed in the case of spinach (Sinios and Wodsak, 1965; Schuphan, 1965; Phillips, 1968b).

The possible production of methemoglobinemia in infants from ingestion of nitrate- or nitrite-containing foods or water has been of great concern in the past, and the subject with various case histories has been reviewed in detail (Bodansky, 1951; Walton, 1951; Steyn, 1960; Phillips, 1968a). Nitrites combine with hemoglobin in the blood thus making it incapable of carrying oxygen. Plants containing large amounts of nitrates have also been reported to cause poisoning of livestock (McIlwain and Schipper, 1963; Sinclair and Jones, 1964). Nitrates in these cases were reduced to nitrites by bacteria before ingestion or in the digestive tract of the animals. Although such reduction of nitrates to nitrites are less likely to occur in healthy human adults this process can take place in the stomach and duodenum of infants under achlorhydric conditions (higher pH) (Phillips, 1968a).

Sodium (or potassium) nitrate and nitrite are permitted as food additives in a number of meat products. The permitted amounts vary in different countries, but in the majority of cases the levels for sodium nitrite lie in the region of 150–500 ppm. In the United States and United Kingdom, the permissible amount of sodium nitrate in the finished products is up to a maximum level of 500 ppm, whereas there is no such upper limit for nitrate in meats sold in Canada and, until recently, this was also the case in the United Kingdom (Canadian Food and Drugs Act and Regulations, 1965; U.S. Food Additive Regulations, C.F.R. 121.1063, 121.1064, 1972; Dehove, 1970; Meijer, 1963; Stenberg et al., 1969; Uhl and Hansen, 1961). The permissible levels of nitrate and nitrite in sausage products have been recently lowered to 3–10 ppm in the USSR (Stenberg et al., 1969).

The addition of nitrate and nitrite serve a dual purpose. Through bacterial reduction of nitrate to nitrite nitric oxide–myoglobin is produced resulting in the production of a stable red color. The nitric oxide–myoglobin complex is converted to a pink pigment called nitric oxide hemochromogen (Fasett, 1966; Watts, 1954). Nitrite, in conjunction with sodium chloride, also acts as a preservative and prevents the outgrowth of harmful bacteria such as *Clostridium botulinum*. The mild thermal processing that is used for curing meats also plays an important role in controlling the outgrowth of bacterial spores (Silliker et al., 1958; Pivnick et al., 1967; Greenberg and Silliker, 1961). Nitrate is slowly reduced to nitrite by the bacteria naturally present in cured meats and the resulting nitrite exhibits a significant inhibitory action on many food-spoiling bacteria. It is interesting to note that some of the bacteria which spoil cured meat products are of the lactobacilli and streptococci types, and these bacteria are also known to be resistant to nitrite

(Ingram, 1959). The reduction of nitrate to nitrite in cured meat products depends on various factors such as temperature, oxygen concentration, supply of hydrogen donors, salt concentration, and the composition and numbers of bacterial flora. The subject has been reviewed recently by Ingram and Dainty (1971).

Although the levels of nitrate and nitrite in cured meat products are strictly controlled, occasionally many commercial products have been found to contain excessive amounts of these chemicals. This may have occurred due to indiscriminate use of these additives or formation of nitrite from nitrate during storage or processing. Orgeron *et al.* (1957) have reported some cases of nitrite poisoning in children that followed the eating of wieners containing 5000 ppm nitrite. Spencer (1970) in the U.K. found high levels of nitrate (up to 1706 ppm) and nitrite (up to 480 ppm) in vacuum-packed bacon. Unusually large amounts of nitrite (1100–2000 ppm) were also reported to be found in vacuum-packed bacon by Eddy and Ingram (1962). Sander (1967a) analyzed a total of 80 samples of meat products (sausages, salami, canned meat) and found an average of 18.5 ppm nitrite. In a recent survey carried out by this laboratory 100 samples of meat products were analyzed and an average of 20.5 ppm sodium nitrite (range, 0–216 ppm) and 255 ppm sodium nitrate (range, 0–3466 ppm) were detected (J. R. Iyengar and T. Panalaks, unpublished data). Although the occurrence of high levels of nitrite in meats is rare, levels in the range of 100 ppm in bacons are quite common (Spencer, 1970).

Sodium nitrate (up to 100 ppm) and sodium nitrite (maximum level, 10 ppm) are allowed in certain types of cheeses in the U.K. (The Preservatives in Food Regulations, HM Stationery Office, London, 1962). Nitrate and/or nitrite are also permitted as preservatives in cheese in the Netherlands, USSR and Sweden (Meijer, 1963; Stenberg *et al.,* 1969; Anonymous, 1969). Nitrate may be added in the following types of cheeses: Danablu, Danbo, Edam, Gouda, Havarti, Jarlsberg, Limburger, Noekkel, Nordbo, Norwegia, Samsoe, Svecia, Steinbuscher, Tilsiter. It is not permitted, however, in the nonmatured cheeses and cheeses of the Cheddar type (Van Ginkel, 1969). Nitrate is believed to prevent butyric acid fermentation in cheese as well as early production of gas from lactose (Galesloot, 1964). However, due to concern about nitrosamine formation such practices are under review at the moment (Van Ginkel, 1969).

Extensive studies by Tarr and Sunderland (1939) showed that sodium nitrite at a concentration of 0.02–0.05%, in combination with sodium chloride (2–20%), retarded bacterial spoilage of fillets of halibut and flounder and increased the keeping quality of stored fish. Such preservative actions of nitrite were highly pH-dependent; suppression of bacterial growth was extremely marked at pH 6, while at pH 7 the retarding effect was negligible (Tarr and Sunderland, 1940a,b). Incorporation of sodium nitrite in ice also proved effective in preventing such spoilage (Tarr and Sunderland, 1940c). Following these successful investigations sodium nitrite was used for some 10–15 years in Canada as a preservative for fish, but later was replaced by chlorotetracycline about 1959 (Tarr, 1969). In northern Norway, a mixture of formalin and sodium nitrite was used for a long time for preserving fish meal, and this practice, as mentioned in the Introduction, precipitated the crisis of fatal liver disease in farm animals due to the formation of DMN in the nitrite-preserved meals.

The U.S. allows the addition of sodium nitrate and sodium nitrite in smoked, cured, sable fish, salmon, shad, and chub. The level of sodium nitrate and sodium nitrite in the final products must be less than 500 and 200 ppm, respectively. The permissible level of sodium nitrite in smoked, cured tuna fish is 10 ppm (U.S. Food Additive Regulations, CFR 121.1063, 121.1064, 121.1230, 1972). Various aspects of the preservation of smoked fish by nitrite have been studied by Weckel and Chien (1969). However, the trend now is to completely eliminate the addition of nitrate and nitrite or reduce their levels in fish and fish meal (Ender et al., 1967). Sweden recently passed legislation banning the use of nitrite for preserving fish, and other countries also are seriously studying the situation (Anonymous, 1969).

In addition to the natural occurrence of nitrate and nitrite in vegetables and their use as food additives these chemicals may contaminate foods during smoking and spray-drying. Manning et al. (1968) have observed that direct gas firing of spray dryers can form up to 13 ppm of nitrate and 3 ppm of nitrite during drying of milk. Small amounts of nitrite have been shown to form during air-drying of potato and corn starch (Gerritsen and De Willigen, 1969). The occurrence of nitrogen oxides in smoke, which is used for preserving fish and meat products, also deserves consideration. Stack gases from fuel oil combustion have been found to contain 1000 ppm nitrogen oxides, and this may have contributed to some extent to the formation of nitrosamines in herring meal implicated in the liver disease of ruminants in Norway (Ender and Ceh, 1967).

B. Amines

Apart from the vast amounts of work published on the occurrence of amines in fish very few data are available as to the presence of various amines in other foods. Although some amino acids and trimethylamine oxide (TMAO) have been shown to produce nitrosamines under unusual conditions, only the secondary and tertiary amines can form nitrosamines in high yields (Ender et al., 1967; Ender and Ceh, 1971). The TMAO content of various fish is important not only because it can produce trace amounts of DMN after treatment with nitrite at high temperature, but also because it is the precursor of trimethylamine (TMA) and dimethylamine (DMA) both of which can easily form DMN on treatment with nitrite.

The distribution and occurrence of TMAO and its metabolites TMA and DMA in fish and other related species have been extensively studied and reviewed elsewhere (Reay and Shewan, 1951; Tomiyasu and Zenitani, 1957). TMAO has been detected in all types of fish except in some molluscus shellfish such as oysters, mussels, or clams (Norris and Benoit, 1945). It is also present in certain types of freshwater fish, although in much smaller quantities than in marine fish (Reay, 1938; Lintzel et al., 1939). Shewan (1951) has reported the occurrence of significant amounts of TMAO in such freshwater fish as the alewife, shad (185 mg%), burbot (116 mg%), salmon (83 mg%), and trout. The elasmobranchs (skate, dogfish, shark, and ray fish) contain the largest amounts. Besides the fish mentioned above the following species also contain considerable amounts of TMAO: herring, clupeids, gadoids, pollack, cod, haddock, hake, cusk, porpoises and whales, shrimp, lobster, crab, and squid (Reay *et al.,* 1943; Sundsvold *et al.,* 1969).

TMA in fish originates from TMAO by bacterial action and the largest amount is naturally found in those which are rich in TMAO. Tarr (1939) demonstrated that the reduction of TMAO to TMA was caused by bacterial enzymes present in the fish. Certain strains of *Micrococcus* and *Achromobacter* were found to reduce TMAO by the action of the enzyme "triaminooxidase" (Tarr, 1940). It was also shown that a variety of oxidizable substrates (lactate, succinate, formate, acetate, fructose, glucose, hexose monophosphate, glycine, and alanine) accelerated this reaction (Tarr, 1939; Watson, 1939).

The presence of large amounts of TMA, which is practically absent in fresh samples of fish has been used as an index of spoilage by various workers (Beatty and Gibbons, 1937; Shewan, 1937a, 1938), and considerable amounts have been detected in samples that had been stored for a long time. In a study involving the examination of more than 100 individual fish (cod, haddock, herring, hake, and pollack) an average of 0.71 mg TMA/100 ml of pressed juice was detected. In spoiled fish this level was found to reach above 40 mg%. Shewan (1937a, 1938) has detected 0–100 mg TMA/100 gm stored haddocks depending on the length of storage. Spoilage odors can be detected by trained observers when the TMA content reaches about 4–6 mg%. Small amounts of TMA have also been detected in partially spoiled or stored elasmobranchs (shark, skate, dogfish) and in squid muscles as well as in fresh squid and in the muscle of various octopi (Borgstrom, 1961).

Many interesting results have been published on the occurrence and formation of DMA in fish. It is usually absent in fresh fish but formed during storage. Shewan (1937b, 1938) first observed its presence in haddock and later found it to be present also in cod, whiting, and herring. It is not formed at all in freshwater perch and dogfish. Recent studies have indicated that the DMA content of several species of gadoid fish (cod, pollack, cusk, hake, and haddock) increases considerably during prolonged storage at freezing temperatures (Tokunga, 1964; Tozawa *et al.,* 1969; Castell *et al.,* 1970, 1971). The largest amount (up to 54 mg%) of DMA was observed to be present in hake after 28 days of storage at

−5°C. Under the same storage conditions no DMA was detected in halibut, plaice, redfish, or wolffish. Large amounts of DMA, as well as TMA, have been detected in the flesh of fish rich in TMAO after γ-irradiation (Amano and Tozawa, 1965). The quantities of DMA formed varied with the species and were highest among the gadoid group; smaller amounts formed in shark and squid. This variation was attributed to the difference in the activity of specific enzymes to split TMAO into DMA and formaldehyde. In addition to the amines mentioned above trace quantities of methyl-, ethyl-, methylethyl-, isopropyl-, diethyl-, n-propyl-, n-butyl-, and isobutylamines have been detected in fish protein concentrates prepared from red hake (Wick et al., 1967). Sarcosine is another nitrosatable amino compound that has been shown to occur in elasmobranch fish (Borgstrom, 1961).

Although it is believed that trace amounts of various amines are present in meat products very little data are available as to the nature and amount of these compounds. Trace amounts of monomethyl-, ethyl-, and n-butylamines have been reported to be present in soured meat sausages but none could be detected in the normal products (Cantoni et al., 1969). Landmann and Batzer (1966) detected methylamine in dry-cured smoked ham, although none could be found in the raw meat. Methylamine and ethylamine are known to be present in irradiated beef (Burks et al., 1959). Both piperidine and pyrrolidine are known to be present in partially decayed meat and fish, and these compounds are produced as metabolites of lysine by bacteria (Saito and Sameshima, 1956). Lijinsky and Epstein (1970) have suggested that cadaverine and putresine can form piperidine and pyrrolidine, respectively, by heat (e.g., during cooking of foods) and to products which may react with nitrite to form the corresponding nitrosamines which are carcinogenic. However, the levels of cadaverine and putresine in normal human diets are so small that these compounds can not be considered as significant contributors of secondary amines (Courts, 1970).

As in the case of meat products only scant information is available on the occurence of secondary and tertiary amines in milk and cheese. Schwarz and Thomasow (1950) reported the presence of methylamine, DMA, and TMA in Tilsiter cheese. Trace amounts of methylamine, DMA, and TMA in *Blauschimmelkaese* (Thomasow, 1947) and of methylamine, DMA, ethylamine and butylamine in milk (Weurman and DeRooy, 1961) have been detected. Recently, the Russian workers (Golovnya *et al.*, 1970) reported the occurrence of a series of amines in Rossiiskii cheese. These workers found approximately 23 and 29.4 mg of total amine hydrochloride mixtures in 500-gm portions of the cheese after maturing for 4 and 6 months, respectively. Methylamine, DMA, diethylamine, dipropylamine, diisopropylamine, dibutylamine, TMA, triethylamine, tripropylamine, piperidine, and α-picoline were among the major amines found. There were considerable variations in the amine compositions with storage time, and these differences reflected the observed deterioration of the flavor score of the cheese during storage.

C. Interaction of Nitrites with Amino Compounds

The reaction of nitrous acid with amines is well known to all organic chemistry students as it is widely used for distinguishing various amines. Nitrite in the presence of strong acids reacts vigorously with primary amines with evolution of nitrogen gas to produce alcohols, olefins, ethers, or alkyl halides depending on the conditions used. Secondary amines, under such conditions, yield nitrosamines which usually separate as a yellowish solid or liquid. Tertiary amines do not react with nitrous acid but remain as salts and can be recovered by the addition of alkali. Although the above statement is generally true, tertiary amines under mildly acidic conditions react with nitrous acid and produce aldehydes and secondary amines which in turn react with nitrous acid and produce the nitrosamines (Roberts and Caserio, 1964; Hein, 1963).

In order to have a wider understanding of the problem of DMN formation in nitrite-preserved herring meal Ender *et al.* (1967) carried out a thorough study of the reaction between nitrite and various methylamines. Methylamine, DMA, TMA, and TMAO all produced DMN when heated with sodium nitrite at various temperatures and pH's. However, the yield varied widely with the conditions and the amines used. DMA was the major contributor; next was TMA. It is interesting to note that monomethylamine, a primary amine, also produced significant amounts of DMN when the reaction mixture was heated for 2 hours at 135°C. The formation of small amounts of DMN from DMA and sodium nitrite took place even under milder conditions (e.g., 2–157 days at 4°C). The amount of DMN formed from DMA and nitrite at pH 6.0 was approximately 2–2.5 times higher than that produced at pH 6.5. In model experiments Malins *et al.* (1970) failed to detect any DMN formation at pH 5.8–6.4 after heating an aqueous mixture of sodium nitrite and TMAO or DMA. Trace amounts (1–8.5 μg) of DMN were, however, detectable in reaction mixtures consisting of 400–2000 ppm TMA and 400 ppm sodium nitrite. From these studies the researchers concluded that commercial processing of smoked chub, a freshwater fish that contains only small amounts of TMA, TMAO, and DMA, with 200 ppm sodium nitrite could not form more than 10 ppb (1 ppb = 10^{-9}) DMN in the final product.

In search for possible precursors of nitrosamines, Devik (1967) studied the reaction between amino acids and aldoses. Lysine, glutamic acid, and alanine were heated with D-glucose and potato starch at different temperatures and pH's. The formation of considerable amounts of nitrosamines was observed especially in the D-glucose/L-alanine heated mixture. The exact nature of the nitrosamines formed were not known, but the TLC and polarographic results indicated the presence of a mixture of nitrosamines, namely, DMN, DEN, and possibly dibutyl-, diamyl-, or dipropylnitrosamines. However, recent works by Heyns and Koch (1970) and Scanlan and Libbey (1971) cast grave doubts on the validity of Devik's results. These workers pointed out that Devik probably misidentified pyrazines and acetylpyrrole, which are products of such reactions, as nitrosamines.

Only recently, it has been established that the reaction between amines and nitrite can take place under the mild conditions that exist in the human stomach. Following the suggestion of Druckrey *et al.* (1963b), Sander (1967a) first demonstrated that certain secondary amines when incubated with human gastric juice and sodium nitrite could form trace amounts of the corresponding nitrosamines. Sander *et al.* (1968) observed that the ease of formation of nitrosamines depends mainly on the basicity of the amines and pH of the reaction mixtures. The weakly basic amines such as diphenylamine, N-methylaniline, morpholine, and N-methylbenzylamine produced the corresponding nitrosamines in high yields, whereas no nitrosamine formation could be detected from the strongly basic amine, diethylamine. The pH optimum for the formation of these nitrosamines was noted to be in the region of 1–3. Sen *et al.* (1969a,b), however, demonstrated that the nitrosation of the strongly basic amine, diethylamine, is possible under conditions similar to that existing in the human stomach. These investigators studied the formation of DEN from diethylamine and sodium nitrite and showed that such a reaction could occur in gastric juices from rats, rabbits, cats, dogs, and man. The amount of DEN produced increased with decrease in pH of the reaction mixture; human and rabbit gastric juices (pH 1–2) produced more DEN than did the rat gastric juice (pH 4–5). The overall yields were very low, and maximum value was only 0.6% of the theoretical. Although the yield of nitrosamine formation from the strongly basic amines (such as DMA, diethylamine) is low, these amines are known to occur in foods in large quantities (Section III,B) and the corresponding nitrosamines are highly carcinogenic. Therefore, the possibility of formation of even trace amounts of these nitrosamines in human stomach cannot be disregarded.

Careful kinetic studies by Mirvish (1970) and others (Taylor and Price, 1929) have established that the rate of nitrosation of DMA is maximal at about pH 3.4 and directly proportional to the concentration of the nonionized amine and the square of the nitrite concentration. Even at the optimum pH the percent yield was only 15.4% of the theoretical. It was concluded that only minute quantities (1–3 μg) of DMN would be expected to form from normal daily dietary intake of DMA and nitrite. However, other chemicals present in the human gastric juice may have considerable influence on the rate of nitrosamine formation and, therefore, the results of the chemical experiments may not be comparable to that occurring under the physiological conditions of human stomach. The report that thiocyanate ions, which are excreted in the human saliva, have a catalytic effect on the nitrosation reaction rate is of particular interest (Boyland *et al.*, 1971). On the other hand, the presence of tannins in the diet may retard such formations (Bogovski *et al.*, 1971).

Sander *et al.* (1971) and Mirvish (1971a,b) have extended the kinetic studies to other nitrosatable compounds such as amino acids, ureas, urethanes, and guanidines. It was demonstrated that the rate of nitrosation depends mainly on the resonance and inductive effects. The alkylureas such as methylurea and ethylurea were most easily nitrosatable, and the reaction rate increased progressively with decrease in pH. Citrulline, a naturally occurring ureido amino acid, produced nitrosocitrulline in good yields. The product from arginine and nitrous acid was believed to be nitrosocitrulline, although convincing evidence for such an assumption was not presented. Nitrite and methylguanidine, which occurs naturally in beef (Komarow, 1929; Kapeller-Adler and Krael, 1930a), shark, rayfish, cod (Kapeller-Adler and Krael, 1930b), and sardine (Sasaki, 1938), produced methylnitrosourea, a potent carcinogen. The amino acids L-proline, L-hydroxyproline, and sarcosine were easily nitrosatable at pH 2.2–2.5, and the nitrosation rate was found to be 140–230 times faster than that of DMA. Since proline and hydroxyproline are components of proteins and large amounts of citrulline occur in various foods (Wada, 1930; Navarro *et al.*, 1962; Ogasawara *et al.*, 1963), the above-mentioned findings will be disturbing if the corresponding nitroso derivatives are found to be carcinogenic. Nitrososarcosine is a strong carcinogen (Druckrey *et al.*, 1967), and the ingestion of large amounts of sarcosine and nitrite in the diet could be a hazard to human health.

Ender and Ceh (1971) investigated the conditions under which various amines, amino acids, and proteins could react with nitrite to form the nitrosamines. As expected, the simple alkylamines, pyrrolidine, and piperidine all produced the corresponding nitrosamines in amounts consistent with the findings discussed above. It is noteworthy that various amino acids such as glycine, valine, and L-alanine also produced nitrosamines (mainly DMN) when heated with sodium nitrite and rice starch (an encapsulating agent) at 130°–170°C (pH 6.0–6.6). In addition to DMN, small amounts of methylethylnitrosamine and DEN were formed from L-alanine. L-Proline produced nitrosopyrrolidine. Similar results were obtained when meat and fish were heated with sodium nitrite and rice starch. These workers pointed out that the level of nitrite used in the study was excessively high (as much as 1.2% in some cases) and, therefore, the production of large amounts of DMN from meat and fish should be regarded as a typical artifact. These workers did not study the formation of nitrosamines in the presence of lower levels of nitrite.

Sen *et al.* (1970) have demonstrated that the cooking process used for preparing meals may influence the formation of nitrosamines. Various fish (cod, herring, hake, halibut, mackerel, and salmon) were treated with 200 ppm sodium nitrite and cooked at 110°C for 60–70 minutes. Trace amounts (2.5–25 ppb) of DMN were detected in the cooked product. Mackerel and hake, both of which are known to contain large amounts of DMA and TMA (Section III,B), produced the largest amounts. The control samples did not contain any detectable nitrosamines. Considerably larger amounts (45 ppb) of DMN were formed when smoked hake was cooked in an autoclave with 200 ppm sodium nitrite for 20 minutes under 20 psi. It was concluded that a 200 ppm residual level of sodium nitrite, if used as an additive, in certain fish could produce nitrosamines under the normal cooking process.

The formation of N-nitroso compounds from foodstuffs, mainly eggs and meats, has been studied by Walters *et al.* (1971). After deliberate nitrosation of these foods with unusually large amounts (1%) of sodium nitrite some indications of the formation of N-nitroso compounds have been observed. The exact nature of the compounds detected is not yet clear.

As cheese contains small amounts of amines (Section III,B) there is a possibility that nitrate-treated cheeses may form nitrosamines. Nitrate is converted to nitrite by the catalytic action of the enzyme xanthine oxidase which is present in milk (Galesloot, 1956). This enzyme is destroyed rapidly in cheese and consequently nitrite disappears from cheese within a few days. Only trace amounts (<10 ppm) of nitrite could be found in cheeses older than 6 weeks (Dubrow and Kabish, 1960; Woerner and Fricker, 1960; Schulz *et al.*, 1960), and in some cases nitrite was undetectable after 4–10 days of storage. Since the amount of amines present in unripened cheeses is negligible there is little likelihood of the concurrent occurrence of amines and nitrite in nitrate-treated cheeses.

Moreover, a major part of the nitrite can be destroyed by reaction with primary amino groups of the cheese proteins thus reducing the chance of the formation of nitrosamines (Van Ginkel, 1969).

D. FORMATION OF NITROSAMINES *IN VIVO*

Results of feeding studies in laboratory animals are in agreement with the chemical *in vitro* findings described in Section III,C. When nitrite and various weakly basic amines such as morpholine, methylbenzylamine, piperazine, or methylaniline were fed to rats or mice high incidence of tumors was observed in the experimental animals (Sander *et al.*, 1968; Greenblatt *et al.*, 1971). Negative results were obtained when the animals received either nitrite or the amines. Although Sen *et al.* (1969b) and Alam *et al.* (1971a,b) have presented strong evidence for the *in vivo* formation of nitrosamines from the strongly basic amines and nitrite, prolonged feeding of DMA, diethylamine, piperidine, or methylacetamide and sodium nitrite failed to induce cancer in rats or mice (Druckrey *et al.*, 1963b; Sander *et al.*, 1968; Greenblatt *et al.*, 1971). It should be pointed out that failure to induce tumors in these cases does not necessarily mean that no nitroso compounds were formed. It is possible that the amount of nitrosamine formed was not sufficient to induce statistically significant number of tumors in the small group of animals tested within the time of the experiment.

Of the amides tested the alkylureas have been shown to be easily nitrosated *in vivo* and to produce tumors in experimental animals. Methylurea, ethylurea, and ethyleneurea (in combination with nitrite) all gave positive results (Sander and Schweinsberg, 1971; Mirvish, 1971a). Feeding experiments on pregnant animals using ethylurea and sodium nitrite induced malignant tumors in the nervous system of the offspring (Ivankovic and Preussmann, 1970). The easiest nitrosatable amide so far tested is ethyleneurea. Concurrent feeding of this compound and sodium nitrite at a concentration of 0.05% each to rats for 156 days produced tumors within 1 year (Sander and Schweinsberg, 1971).

Recent studies (Sander, 1968; Sander and Seif, 1969; Klubes and Jondrof, 1971; Hawksworth and Hill, 1971) indicate that certain bacteria can synthesize nitrosamines from secondary amines and nitrate or nitrite. Certain species of streptococci and *Escherichia coli* were found to be very active in this respect. Increased synthesis was observed in the presence of glucose. Highest yields of nitrosamines were obtained from the weakly basic amine, diphenylamine. Since the level of nitrate and nitrite in human large bowel is negligible, the investigators Hill and Hawksworth (1971) concluded that there is little risk of formation of nitrosamines by bacteria. However, the case of urinary tract infection, mainly by *E. coli*, is quite common and under these circumstances nitrosamines could be produced in the bladder.

As many foods contain amines, nitrate and nitrite, the microorganisms present in these foods may play an important role in the synthesis of nitrosamines in foods. Lembke and Moebus (1970) have investigated such possibilities and examined the role of microorganisms in the formation of nitrosamines in cheese. A nitrite-producing organism, *Micrococcus conglomeratus*, was found to be associated with a cheese containing some nitrosamine. The identity and the amount of the nitrosamine found were not reported. Nitrite-producing organisms were reported to prevail mostly in the outer layer of the cheeses examined. There did not seem to be any relation between the nitrate-producing organism and the nitrosamine contents.

IV. Occurrence

A. Fish and Fish Meal

As mentioned in the Introduction the first evidence for the presence of DMN in food or feed came from the study of Ender *et al.* (1964) investigating the liver disease in ruminants. Preliminary studies pointed out that this disorder occurred in livestock which were fed nitrite-preserved herring meal produced by a single factory in northern Norway (Koppang, 1964). The toxic factor was more concentrated in the meal that was processed immediately after the addition of nitrite, and more was formed when the meal was processed at 115–130°C than at 40°C. Extraction of the toxic factor from the dry meal proved difficult as it was insoluble in ether, chloroform, and acetone, and aqueous extraction methods produced nontoxic extracts. An attempt was made to isolate the "mother-substances" which in turn could be reacted with nitrite to produce the toxic compound. Rice starch was added to the "mother-substances" to avoid loss of the toxic factor. Large amounts of the "mother-substances" were isolated from the skin of herring and cod and finally identified to be aliphatic amines, mainly DMA and TMA. This discovery clearly suggested the formation of DMN which was shown to produce pathological symptoms in mink similar to that caused by the toxic meal. Subsequent studies by Sakshaug *et al.* (1965) confirmed the presence of large amounts of DMN in the toxic herring meal. The concentration of DMN in six of these feeds ranged from 30 to 100 ppm. Two of the three other suspected samples contained 15 and 40 ppm DMN and one contained none. No DMN could be detected in six batches of nontoxic herring meal. Thin-layer chromatography (TLC) was used for the detection and semiquantitative estimation of DMN (detection limit, 10–15 ppm). The temperature used for drying the meal, the concentration of sodium nitrite, and the interval between nitrite treatment and subsequent processing by heat controlled the DMN content of the final product (Ender, 1966; Ender *et al.*, 1967; Koppang and Helgebostad, 1966).

Ender and Ceh (1967) also carried out investigations on the nitrosamine contents of smoked fish used for human consumption. Trace amounts (0.5–40 ppb) of DMN were detected in smoked herring, haddock, mackerel, and kippers. All of the 12 samples analyzed gave positive tests for nitrosamines. Using a sensitive gas–liquid chromatographic (GLC) method (detection limit 10 ppb) Howard *et al.* (1970) analyzed five experimental lots of smoked nitrite-treated chub fish but could not detect any DMN in these samples. However, in a more recent study these workers (Fazio *et al.*, 1971a) have reported the presence of a 4–26 ppb DMN in some smoked marine fish. DMN was found in all of the 15 samples of sable analyzed; the raw unprocessed products contained the lowest amounts (4 ppb), whereas the smoked and nitrate (or nitrite)-treated smoked samples contained considerably more (up to 14 ppb). Two lots of smoked sable, which were treated with both nitrate and nitrite, were found to contain 20 and 26 ppb DMN, respectively. Smoked, nitrate–nitrite-treated salmon and shad contained 4–17 ppb DMN. No DMN was detected in the raw unprocessed salmon and shad. These findings confirm earlier observations by Sen *et al.* (1970) that the treatment of marine fish with 200 ppm sodium nitrite may result in the formation of nitrosamines in the final product (Section III,C).

B. MEAT

The earliest report of the occurrence of nitrosamine in meat was published by Ender and Ceh (1967). Trace amounts of DMN were detected in 3 smoked sausages (0.8–2.4 ppb), 2 bacons (0.6–6.5 ppb), and 1 smoked ham (5.7 ppb). While studying the effect of nitrite on the formation of nitrosamines in meat products, Moehler and Mayrhofer (1969) observed the presence of 5 ppb DEN in an uncooked sausage and the same amount of di-*n*-propylnitrosamine in each of a sample of cured meat, and a cured, smoked, pork belly. Both of these products contained a residual level of 10 ppm nitrite in each case. About 5 ppb of each of DEN and di-*n*-propylnitrosamine were also detected in canned ribs containing 50 ppm nitrite. These investigators concluded that trace amounts of nitrosamines with short alkyl chains may occur in meats if the nitrite content is 10 ppm or more. No nitrosamines could be detected in the untreated (with nitrate or nitrite) meat. In an earlier study, however, these workers (Moehler and Mayrhofer, 1968) reported the occurrence of 0.25 ppm DMN in a sample of raw untreated beef. Recently, Freimuth and Glaeser (1970) have found up to 40 ppb DEN in cured meat products (Kasseler ribs).

Sen (1972) has carried out an extensive investigation of the volatile nitrosamine contents of various meat products. Altogether 59 samples (bacon; corned beef; canned meat; smoked beef, ham, and pork; smoked sausages; and salami) were analyzed, and approximately 10–80 ppb DMN were detected in 5 samples of sausages or salami. All other samples were negative. Fairly large amounts of an unknown compound, which was indistinguishable from DEN by the TLC test, were detected in 4 sausages, but the compound behaved differently on GLC analysis. The identity of this compound is under investigation. Strong TLC evidence has been obtained for the presence of about 10 ppb nitrosopyrrolidine in a sample of cooked bacon (N. P. Sen, unpublished data).

Fazio *et al.* (1971b), in the U.S., analyzed 51 samples of various meat products, and only 1 of them (a smoked ham) was found to contain 5 ppb DMN. Other samples analyzed consisted of the following types of meats: cold cuts; sausages; baby foods; canned meats; bacon, ham, and other pork products; miscellaneous beef products. Many of these samples gave positive indications of the presence of 2–3 ppb DMN, but, because of experimental difficulties, these workers did not attempt to confirm these low positive results by GLC–mass spectrometry. In a similar study, Fiddler *et al.* (1971) did not find any DMN in 10 samples of ham analyzed in their laboratory. Telling *et al.* (1971) in the U.K. also failed to detect any nitrosamine in 7 types of meat products analyzed by a method that is sensitive to 25–65 ppb of volatile nitrosamines.

C. CHEESE

The data so far published on the nitrosamine content in various cheeses are very meager, and convincing evidence of their presence in cheese is yet to be presented. Kroeller (1967) examined 22 samples of Tilsit cheese and 30 Dutch cheese and detected trace amounts (5–10 ppb) of di-*n*-propylnitrosamine or diisopropylnitrosamine in one Havarti and one Gouda cheese. Some of the Tilsit cheese analyzed were prepared by adding saltpeter, but these samples as well as all other samples were negative. The investigator was unable to make clear distinction between the two nitrosamines. It is, therefore, not certain which of the aforementioned nitrosamines were present in the two positive samples. Sen *et al.* (1969a) failed to get conclusive evidence of any nitrosamine in 6 samples of cheddar cheese analyzed.

Evidence for the presence of fairly large amounts (0.12 ppm) of DMN in a Tollenser cheese has been reported (Freimuth and Glaeser, 1970). Another sample of the same cheese contained trace

TABLE I

Reported Occurrence of Nitrosamines in Animal Foodstuffs

Kind	Country of origin	Nitrosamines found	Levels	Method[a] used	References
Fish and Fish Meal					
Herring meal	Norway	DMN	15–100 ppm	TLC, GLC, IR, UV	Sakshaug et al. (1965); Ender et al. (1964)
Fish Meal	Canada	DMN	0.35–0.5 ppm	TLC, GLC GLC–MS	N. P. Sen (unpublished data)
Smoked herring, haddock, mackerel and kippers	Norway and Iceland	DMN	0.5–40 ppb	TLC and colorimetric	Ender and Ceh (1967)
Smoked, nitrate/or nitrite treated sable, salmon and shad	U.S.A.	DMN	4–26 ppb	GLC, GLC–MS	Fazio et al. (1971a)
Salt-dried fish	Hong Kong	DMN and DEN	0.6–21 ppm	TLC, GLC	Fong and Walsh (1971)
Meat Products					
Smoked sausage	Norway	DMN	0.8–2.4 ppb	TLC and colorimetric	Ender and Ceh (1967)
Bacon	Norway	DMN	0.6–6.5 ppb	TLC and colorimetric	Ender and Ceh (1967)
Smoked ham	Norway	DMN	5.7 ppb	TLC and colorimetric	Ender and Ceh (1967)
Uncooked sausage	Germany	DEN	5 ppb	TLC	Moehler and Mayrhofer (1969)
Cured, smoked, pork belly	Germany	Di-n-propyl-nitrosamine	5 ppb	TLC	Moehler and Mayrhofer (1969)
Canned ribs	Germany	DEN and Di-n-propylnitros-amine	5 ppb	TLC	Moehler and Mayrhofer (1969)
Raw untreated beef	Germany	DMN	0.25 ppm	TLC, GLC	Moehler and Mayrhofer (1968)

	Country	Nitrosamine	Amount	Method	Reference
Cured meat (Kasseler ribs)	Germany	DEN	Trace–40 ppb	TLC	Freimuth and Glaeser (1970)
Dry sausage	Canada	DMN	10–20 ppb	TLC, GLC GLC–MS	Sen (1972)
Uncooked salami	Canada	DMN	20–80 ppb	TLC, GLC GLC–MS	Sen (1972)
Cooked bacon	Canada	Nitroso-pyrrolidine	10 ppb	TLC	N. P. Sen (unpublished data)
Smoked ham	U.S.A.	DMN	5 ppb	GLC, GLC–MS	Fazio et al. (1971b)
Cheese and Milk					
Havarti cheese ⎱ Gouda cheese ⎰	Germany	Diisopropylnitrosamine and/or Di-n-propyl-nitrosamine	5–10 ppb	TLC, GLC	Kroeller (1967)
Tollenser cheese	Germany	DMN	0.12 ppm	TLC	Freimuth and Glaeser (1970)
Tollenser cheese	Germany	DEN	Trace	TLC	Freimuth and Glaeser (1970)
Cheese	Germany	Unidentified nitrosamine	Unspecified	Colorimetric	Lembke and Moebus (1970)
Cheese	Germany	DEN	Unspecified	TLC, GLC	Hedler and Marquardt (1968)
Cheese	Germany	DEN	Unspecified	TLC, GLC	Hedler and Marquardt (1968)
Pasteurized milk	Germany	DEN	Unspecified	TLC	Hedler and Marquardt (1968)

[a]See Section V for abbreviations.

157

amounts of DEN but no DMN. Altogether 6 samples of Tollenser, 3 Gouda, and 2 Edam cheeses were analyzed in this study, and the rest of the samples were negative.

Van Ginkel (1969) studied the effect of nitrate on the nitrosamine content of Edam cheese. Cheese was prepared by the usual technique with or without the addition of potassium nitrate; two levels (200 and 400 ppm) of potassium nitrate were used. The samples were analyzed for nitrate, nitrite and nitrosamines after varying periods (6–12 weeks) of storage. It was concluded that only small amounts (<0.1 ppm) of nitrosamines, if any, were present in these samples, and the data did not correlate at all with the nitrate and nitrite content or age of the cheese. Thirty samples of Dutch cheese (Gouda and Edam) were also analyzed, but no nitrosamines could be detected. Lembke and Moebus (1970) analyzed 77 semihard and soft cheeses; the nitrosamines found were less than 0.2 ppm. No information as to the nature of the nitrosamine detected was presented.

Table I summarizes the data published so far on the occurrence of nitrosamines in animal foodstuffs. The methods used for determining nitrosamines in many cases are very nonspecific and, therefore, the results should be interpreted with caution. To emphasize this point, information about the method used in various cases is also included in the table.

D. OTHER FOODS

Marquardt and Hedler (1966) in Germany published a paper describing the finding of DEN in wheat flour. By using a TLC method, these workers found rather large amounts of DEN, especially after heating the flour for 7 hours at 170°C. No quantitative estimations were made, but a level of 50 ppm was suggested. Thewlis (1967, 1968) in England strongly disputed these findings and suggested that the TLC test used by Marquardt and Hedler (1966) was nonspecific and the positive results could have resulted from interfering phenolic substances which are present in flour. Hedler and Marquardt (1968) reiterated their previous claim and reported the presence of DEN in wheat flour, as well as in wheat plant, and wheat grain. These workers also detected DEN in one sample of flour provided by Thewlis. Kroeller (1967) also investigated the nitrosamine contents of commercial samples of wheat flour and reported finding 10 ppb DEN in 1 out of 30 samples analyzed. Moehler and Mayrhofer (1968) detected 0.3 ppm DMN in a flour sample, but Sen *et al.* (1969a) failed to detect any nitrosamines in flour, even after heating the samples for 6 hours at 150°–160°C.

Similar controversy exists with regard to the occurrence of nitrosamines in distilled spirits. The publication of the finding of DMN or nitrosamine-like compounds in African alcoholic spirits by McGlashan *et al.* (1968) and McGlashan and Walters (1969) aroused a great deal of interest because of the implication of linking high incidence of esophageal cancer in African natives to the consumption of these locally distilled alcoholic drinks. The levels of DMN detected in these samples were quite high and ranged between 1.5 and 6.0 ppm. However, these researchers were not definite as to the identity of the compounds involved and further research was being continued to characterize the components that behaved like *N*-nitrosamines on polarographic analysis. In a recent communication by McGlashan *et al.* (1970) it was pointed out that the polarographic technique used in the above-mentioned studies is nonspecific and interference can be obtained from furfural which is a natural constituent of many alcoholic beverages. Sen and Dalpé (1972) have been unable to detect any nitrosamines in alcoholic beverages.

The high incidence of esophageal cancer in Bantu people in the Transkei region in South Africa prompted DuPlessis *et al.* (1969) to search for possible carcinogens in the diet of the African natives. The first positive result indicated the presence of DMN in the fruit of a solanaceous bush, *Solanum incanum,* the juice of which is used for curdling milk. These investigators carried out an extensive analysis of the compound isolated from the fruit, and identified it as DMN on the basis of TLC, GLC, and infrared and nuclear magnetic resonance spectroscopic data. Although no information was presented as to the exact level of DMN, it appears from their results that at least 1 mg DMN was isolated from 4.3 kg of the fruit.

The precursors necessary for the formation of nitrosamines occur in tobacco and, therefore, it is likely that tobacco or tobacco smoke may contain trace amounts of nitrosamines (Druckrey and Preussmann, 1962b). But initial searches for nitrosamines in tobacco products have been hampered due to experimental difficulties. Nevertheless, evidence for the presence of DMN, nitrosopyrrolidine, methylbutylnitrosamine, and nitrosopiperidine in tobacco smoke has been obtained (Neurath *et al.*, 1964; Serfontein and Hurter, 1966; Kroeller, 1967; Neurath, 1971). Although anabasine and nornicotine are constituents of tobacco smoke, the corresponding nitroso derivatives were not detected (Neurath, 1971).

There are only two reports in the literature of the occurrence of nitrosamines in mushrooms. The first report from Germany (Herrmann, 1961) presented evidence for the isolation and characterization of a compound identical to *p*-methylnitrosaminobenzaldehyde from an edible mushroom, *Clitocybe suaveolens*. Later works by Druckrey *et al.* (1967) and Herrmann *et al.* (1966) have shown that this compound is devoid of any carcinogenic activity. In a more recent study Ender and Ceh (1967) have found trace amounts of DMN in edible mushrooms. Altogether 11 samples (various types) were analyzed, and all contained some DMN (average level 10 ppb); one sample of *Amanita muscaria* contained as much as 30 ppb DMN. The presence of DMN in these mushrooms was attributed to the occurrence of methylamines in mushrooms and interaction with nitrite which was derived from the soil.

As spinach contains large amounts of nitrate and sometimes nitrite (Section III,A) it was thought that nitrosamines could be present in this vegetable. However, only negative results have so far been reported (Sen *et al.*, 1969a; Keybets *et al.*, 1970). Recent reports (Hedler *et al.*, 1971) indicate that soybean oil may contain fairly large amounts of DMN (0.45 ppm) and dibutylnitrosamine (0.29 ppm). The identity of DMN was confirmed by GLC–mass spectrometry.

V. Methods for Identification and Quantitative Estimation

The detection of nitrosamines in foods, especially at parts per billion levels, is a lengthy and tedious process, and there are no simple reliable methods available at the moment. The entire process of analytical methodology can be divided into three major steps: extraction and distillation from foods; purification; and qualitative and quantitative determination. The cleanup procedures described in this section are only applicable to the volatile nitrosamines. Unfortunately, no satisfactory method is available at the moment for determining nonvolatile nitrosamines in foods, although some progress has been made in this area. Some of these techniques will be discussed in subsection D.

A. EXTRACTION AND DISTILLATION

Various methods have been used to separate the nitrosamines from foods, although most of them are quite similar. All of these methods take advantage of the fact that many of the nitrosamines are steam-volatile and can be effectively separated from the majority of food constituents by steam distillation from alkaline, neutral, or acidic solutions (Heath and Jarvis, 1955). However, to prevent the formation of nitrosamines as artifacts all nitrites should be removed or destroyed before subjecting the sample to distillation from an acidic solution (Sen *et al.*, 1970; Eisenbrand *et al.*, 1970a).

Other workers (Kroeller, 1967; Sen *et al.*, 1969a) favor extraction of the nitrosamines from foods into suitable solvents prior to distillation. Due to their high volatility methylene chloride and diethylether are considered most suitable for this purpose. The addition of potassium carbonate solution to the food matrix produces a better release of nitrosamines, and has been reported to give improved recoveries from some foods, especially cheeses (Sen *et al.*, 1969a). Howard *et al.* (1970) first digested their fish samples with methanolic potassium hydroxide for 8 hours before subjecting the samples to distillation. Walters (1971) and Crosby *et al.* (1971) observed that volatile nitrosamines can be effectively distilled in a small volume of liquid by codistillation with methanol or ethanol. Telling *et al.* (1971) obtained improved recoveries of nitrosamines, especially high molecular weight dialkylnitrosamines and some of the heterocyclic *N*-nitrosamines, by vacuum distillation.

B. Purification

There are three cleanup techniques described in the literature based on ion exchange resins (Sen *et al.*, 1969a,b), basic alumina (Sen *et al.*, 1970), and acid–Celite (Howard *et al.*, 1970) column chromatography. Aqueous solutions of nitrosamines (pH 4.5) can be passed through a cation-exchange resin column, Amberlite CG-120, and recovered in the eluate. Sen *et al.* (1969b) also used an anion-exchange resin (Amberlite IRA-400) for selectively removing nitrite from an alkaline (pH 10) solution of nitrosamine and employed the technique for studying the formation of nitrosamines in human and animal gastric juices (Section III,C). However, dialkylnitrosamines with a carbon number greater than 8 as well as nitrosopyrrolidine could not be analyzed due to excessive losses on the resin column (Telling *et al.*, 1971; Sen, 1971).

Sen *et al.* (1970) later used a basic alumina column for cleanup of food extracts and reported much improved results. Howard *et al.* (1970) used an acidified Celite column as a cleanup step for the analysis of meat and fish for DMN. The technique was, however, found unsuitable for the analysis of high molecular weight nitrosamines. To overcome this difficulty, these workers (Fazio *et al.*, 1971c) replaced the Celite with a silica gel column and successfully applied the technique for the analysis of a series of dialkylnitrosamines as well as nitrosopyrrolidine.

In order to separate as selectively as possible both volatile and nonvolatile nitrosamines Walters and his associates (1970, 1971) have used a property which is common to both kinds of nitrosamines, namely, adsorption on activated charcoals. Volatile nitrosamines were separated by steam distillation, and the residual charcoal was used for the analysis of nonvolatile nitrosamines. Since lipids interfere with the adsorption of nitrosamines on charcoal, this technique may not be applicable to food samples that are rich in fats or lipids. Eisenbrand *et al.* (1970b) described a technique whereby various nitrosamines could be separated by gel chromatography on Sephadex LH-20, but, due to interferences from other compounds the technique could not be applied to biological materials.

As some of the nitrosamines, especially low molecular weight dialkylnitrosamines, are highly volatile care should be taken to avoid losses of the compounds during concentration to small volumes. The use of Kuderna-Danish evaporator has been shown to give satisfactory results (Eisenbrand *et al.*, 1970c; Howard *et al.*, 1970; Telling *et al.*, 1971). It is possible to concentrate such solutions to as low as 0.5 ml with the help of a Micro Snyder column and obtain 90% recoveries (Sen and Dalpé, 1972).

C. ESTIMATION

A wide variety of methods have been used for the qualitative and quantitative determination of nitrosamines. These include ultraviolet (Moehler and Mayrhofer, 1968; Daiber and Preussmann, 1964; Ender *et al.*, 1964), infrared spectroscopic (Moehler and Mayrhofer, 1968; Rao, 1963; Levin *et al.*, 1970); fluorometric (Moehler and Mayrhofer, 1968); polarographic; colorimetric; TLC; GLC; and combined GLC–mass spectrometric methods. The first three of these methods are unsuitable for the analysis of foods mainly because of the lack of sensitivity and specificity. The chromatographic techniques are more sensitive and specific, and, because of this, they have been widely used by various investigators. Excellent progress has recently been made on GLC analysis of nitrosamines, and, with the introduction of combined GLC–mass spectrometry, it is now possible to make unequivocal confirmation of nitrosamines at ppb levels. Heath and Jarvis (1955) first applied the polarographic technique to determine DMN in animal tissues. Recently, other workers (Devik, 1967; McGlashan *et al.*, 1968; Walters *et al.*, 1970) have extended the scope of the technique and measured nitrosamines in a variety of materials. The method is quite sensitive, and, with hydrochloric acid as the supporting solvent, a 0.05 ppm level of some nitrosamines can be detected.

The most sensitive colorimetric method so far reported is that described by Daiber and Preussmann (1964) in which the nitrosamines are cleaved to nitrite under weakly alkaline conditions by the action of UV light (short wave). The liberated nitrite is determined with Griess reagent (Sander, 1967b; Walters, 1971). In the technique of Eisenbrand and Preussmann (1970) nitrosamines are quantitatively decomposed to nitrosyl bromide and secondary amines, and the liberated NO^+ ion is coupled with N-[napthyl-(1)]-ethylenediamine to produce a colored solution. The technique was applied to a series of 17 nitrosamines, and, except in the case of methylvinylnitrosamine (92.8% yield), an average recovery of 99.5% was reported.

Because of the simplicity and inexpensive nature of the TLC technique it is very popular among the analysts. Most of the procedures are based on that described by Preussmann et al. (1964a,b). The sensitivity is 0.5–2 μg depending on the nitrosamines used. Preussmann et al. (1964b) used a mixture of sulfanilic acid and 1-napthylamine (Griess reagent) as the second spray reagent. In addition to these reagents Kroeller (1967) and Sen et al. (1969a) used ninhydrin solution as a reagent for detection. The reaction is based on the splitting of nitrosamines under UV light at an acid pH and subsequent detection of the liberated amines with ninhydrin. Organic nitrites, C-nitroso compounds, and free amines, although rarely present in purified food extracts, give positive tests with Griess or ninhydrin reagents usually without UV irradiation. However, these compounds can be easily differentiated from the nitrosamines by the fact that the latter give positive tests only after irradiation. A positive reaction to both the ninhydrin and Griess reagents can be considered as an indication of the presence of nitrosamines.

Nitrosamines can be reduced to hydrazines and then detected by TLC after the formation of suitable derivatives (Neurath et al., 1964; Serfontein and Hurter, 1966). Eisenbrand (1971) has reported a method which depends on the liberation of secondary amines from nitrosamines and determination of the amines by TLC as the highly fluorescent dansyl (1-dimethylaminonapthalene-5-sulfonyl) derivatives. Sen and Dalpé (1972) have pointed out that the TLC analysis of both the parent nitrosamines as well as the nitramine derivatives is useful as it provides additional confirmation. R_f values of the nitramine derivatives are usually higher than that of the nitrosamines.

GLC provides a very sensitive tool for the analysis of nitrosamines. Much of the early work was carried out with pure nitro-

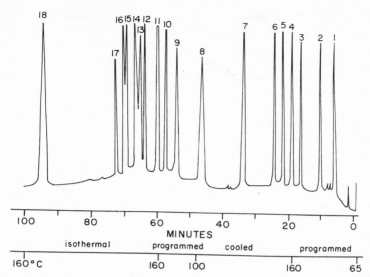

Fig. 2. Separation of nitrosamines by capillary gas chromatography (reproduced from Heyns and Roeper (1970), Copyright, Pergamon Press Ltd.). (1) DMN, (2) DEN, (3), diisopropylnitrosamine, (4) *n*-propylisopropylnitrosamine, (5) di-*n*-propylnitrosamine, (6) ethyl-*n*-butylnitrosamine, (7) diisobutylnitrosamine, (8) *n*-pentylethylnitrosamine, (9) *sec*-butyl-*n*-butylnitrosamine, (10) *n*-pentylisopropyl-nitrosamine, (11) di-*n*-butylnitrosamine, (12) *n*-pentyl-*n*-propylnitrosamine, (13) *n*-pentyl-*sec*-butylnitrosamine, (14) diisopentylnitrosamine, (15) *n*-pentyl-*n*-butylnitro-samine, (16) *n*-pentylisopentylnitrosamine, (17) di-*n*-pentylnitrosamine, and (18) di-*n*-hexylnitrosamine.

samine standards using hydrogen flame ionization and thermal conductivity detectors as the sensing device (Kroeller, 1967; Petrowitz, 1968; Moehler and Mayrhofer, 1968). The cleanup procedures available at that time were not suitable for trace analysis of nitrosamines in foods. Sen *et al.* (1969a, 1970) described a GLC technique for the identification of nitrosamines isolated from foods. Carbowax 20M, Reoplex 400, and SE-30 were used as liquid phases in these studies.

Since it is theoretically possible to have a number of nitrosamines in the same mixture, an ideal method should be capable of distinguishing all of these compounds. In an attempt to separate as many nitrosamines as possible on single GLC columns various workers have investigated different liquid phases. Heyns and Roeper (1970) succeeded in resolving 18 dialkylnitrosamines, some of which are closely related isomers, on a 25-m alkalized polypropylene glycol capillary column (Fig. 2). Foreman *et al.* (1970) used a 6 ft × 1/8 in. stainless steel column packed with Chromosorb 101 (porous polymers) and obtained good separations of 6 alkylnitrosamines. Sen (1970) has provided a method in which nitrosamines are oxidized to nitramines and then detected by GLC using an electron capture detector. The method proved to be extremely sensitive, and about 16 pg of DMN could be detected. Althorpe *et al.* (1970) reported a similar method and extended it to the analysis of a few other nitrosamines. In another method (Eisenbrand, 1971) the amines liberated from the nitrosamines were converted to heptafluorobutyryl derivatives and then analyzed by GLC using an electron capture detector.

Scientists have attempted to improve the specificity of the GLC methods by using nitrogen-specific detectors (Howard *et al.*, 1970; Fiddler *et al.*, 1971). Rhoades and Johnson (1970) have reported that the Coulson Electrolytic Conductivity detector, when used in the pyrolytic mode, is highly specific for nitrosamines. Only amines and those nitrosamines which produce amines under the pyrolytic conditions are detected. For some nitrosamines (e.g., nitrosopyrrolidine) the reductive mode is used whereby these compounds are first reduced to ammonia and then detected. Other workers (Crosby *et al.*, 1971; Issenberg and Tannenbaum, 1971; Sen, 1971) have used the technique for the analysis of foods and found it extremely useful. N. P. Sen and T. Panalaks (unpublished data) obtained 80–90% recoveries of DMN and DEN when added to meat products at 10–20 ppb levels. This appears to be the simplest and most specific method available at the moment for determining volatile nitrosamines in foods.

Various methods for determining nitrosamines so far described are useful for carrying out preliminary analysis of foods, but any positive results obtained cannot be considered as final proof of the identity of the compounds. Due to their carcinogenic nature it is imperative that their identities be unequivocally established. Heyns and Roeper (1970) described a sophisticated GLC–mass spectrometric technique for final confirmation. The combination of capillary column gas chromatography with a fast-scanning mass spectrometer (ATLAS, CH4) allowed unequivocal identification of various nitrosamines. The detection limit of the mass spectrometer was in the region of 0.01 μg per compound. Other workers (Howard et al., 1970; Telling et al., 1971; Sen, 1972) have used similar techniques for detecting nitrosamines in foods.

Most of the volatile nitrosamines produced characteristic mass spectra and exhibit a strong molecular (M^+) ion peak. Collin (1954) has examined a series of dialkylnitrosamines and was able to establish the composition of the most abundant ions. The nitric oxide ion (m/e 30), which is produced from the nitroso group, is always of low-medum abundance. With high molecular weight dialkylnitrosamines an α-cleavage of one alkyl chain occurs followed by a further loss of HNO (Budzikiewicz et al., 1967). Thus, the mass spectrum of di-n-propylnitrosamine contains a peak due to $CH_3-CH_2-CH_2-N^+ \equiv CH$ (m/e 70). A peak corresponding to m/e 27 is believed to be due to hydrogen cyanide. Most of the nitrosamines, except DMN, show a prominent peak at $M - 17$ due to elimination of an hydroxyl radical. Di-n-propylnitrosamine also exhibits a strong peak at m/e 42 which has been assigned the structure $CH_2=N^+=CH_2$. For DMN the strongest peak is the molecular ion peak at m/e 74 followed by two major fragments of composition $M-HNO$ and $M-H_2NO$ corresponding to m/e 43 and 42, respectively. Many nitrosamines undergo a cleavage at C-N bond with the formation of alkyl ions and their degradation products.

D. PROBLEMS IN THE ANALYSIS OF NONVOLATILE NITROSAMINES

Unfortunately, the nonvolatile nitrosamines cannot be steam-distilled, and the cleanup procedures available at the moment are not adequate for trace analysis. Walters et al. (1970) showed that these compounds can be purified by the charcoal adsorption technique described earlier (Section V,B), and then determined polarographically. However, the experiments were carried out with pure standards only and not applied to any foods. The liquid–liquid distribution technique of Eisenbrand et al. (1969) can be used as part of the cleanup procedures and colorimetric techniques employed for end determination. Liquid chromatography or GLC, after suitable derivative formation, may be useful, but considerable research is needed before satisfactory methods will be available for these compounds.

VI. Biological Actions

Various aspects of the biological action of nitrosamines have been reviewed in detail elsewhere (Magee and Schoental, 1964; Magee and Barnes, 1967; Druckrey et al., 1967, 1969; Magee and Swann, 1969; Magee, 1969, 1971). Therefore, only certain findings particularly relevant to this review will be discussed. The reader is advised to consult the above-mentioned references for a more comprehensive survey.

A. ACUTE AND SUBACUTE TOXICITY

The suspicion that DMN could cause acute or subacute poisoning and cirrhosis in men working with this compound led Barnes and Magee (1954) to investigate its toxic properties. In this important study, these workers reported that DMN in doses 20–40 mg/kg produced severe liver damage in rats, rabbits, mice, guinea pigs, and dogs, and all the animals eventually died. A single dose of 25 mg/kg, whether given orally or intraperitoneally, produced similar symptoms in rats. Mice and rabbits were more susceptible; a dose of 10–20 mg/kg proved lethal. Pathological examination revealed hemorrhagic centrilobular necrosis in the liver with a sharp demarcation between the damaged and undamaged liver tissue. Severe gastrointestinal hemorrhage and hemorrhage into the peritoneal cavity was observed in dogs, rats, and guinea pigs treated with DMN. Impaired renal function was also noted in rabbits, but no structural changes, apart from vascular congestion, were observed (O'Leary et al., 1957).

Other nitrosamines produced toxic signs in laboratory animals including liver damage, hemorrhagic lung lesions, convulsions, and coma. The acute oral LD_{50} values of several nitroso compounds are listed in Table II. It should be noted that there appears to

TABLE II
Acute Toxicity of Nitroso Compounds[a]

Compound	Dose (mg/kg)
DMN	27–41
DEN	216
Di-*n*-butylnitrosamine	1200
Methyl-*n*-butylnitrosamine	130
Methyl-*tert*-butylnitrosamine	700
Di-*n*-amylnitrosamine	1750
Methylphenylnitrosamine	200
Methylbenzylnitrosamine	18
Ethyl-*iso*-propylnitrosamine	1100
Ethyl-*n*-butylnitrosamine	380
Ethyl-*tert*-butylnitrosamine	1600
Ethylvinylnitrosamine	88
Ethyl-2-hydroxyethylnitrosamine	> 7500
Di-2-hydroxyethylnitrosamine	> 5000
n-Butyl-4-hydroxybutylnitrosamine	1800
Nitrosomorpholine	282
Nitrososarcosine	> 4000
Nitrososarcosine ethyl ester	> 5000
N,N'-Dinitroso-*N,N'*-dimethylethylenediamine	150
Nitrosomethylurea	180
Nitrosomethylurethane	240
Nitrosotrimethylurea	250

[a]All figures are for single oral LD_{50} dose for rats (Reproduced from Magee and Barnes, 1967), Copyright, Academic Press, Inc.

be no correlation between acute toxicity and carcinogenicity of the nitrosamines. The acute toxicity of DMN, for example, is about eight times that of DEN in rats, but the latter is equally, if not more, active as a liver carcinogen.

Barnes and Magee (1954) studied the effect of chronic feeding of diets containing 50, 100, and 200 ppm DMN to rats. All rats fed DMN at the 200 ppm level died or were killed *in extremis* within 34–37 days. Although there was no gross peritoneal exudate, some evidence of hemorrhage was observed in the gut. The retroperitoneal and retrosternal lymph glands appeared red. The liver was small, and there were obvious signs of fibrosis, especially in those rats dying in the later stages of the experiment. The rats receiving the medium level of DMN died after 62–95 days. All had signs of decreased body weight gains as compared to the control rats. The rats in the last two groups were severely emaciated. All the rats in the first group survived, but the mean weight was significantly lower than that of the controls.

The liver is the major organ affected by acute or subacute doses of nitrosamines. In the majority of cases, necrosis is restricted to the centrilobular area, although generalized necrosis of the liver has been observed in the hamster (Carter *et al.*, 1969). Carlton and Wesler (1968) have reported the development of lesions and sclerosis of the kidney after feeding 0.005% DMN for 8 weeks to Pekin ducks. DMN is more toxic to sheep and fur-bearing animals than to laboratory animals. A single dose of 5 mg/kg or 12 consecutive daily doses of 0.5 mg/kg body weight in sheep can be very toxic and sometimes lethal (Sakshaug *et al.*, 1965). The most common signs are anorexia, absence of ruminal movement, dullness, ataxia of the hind limbs, and frequent respiration. When cows received more than 0.1 mg DMN/kg body weight/day, pronounced hepatotoxic effects were noticeable after 1–6 months. However, daily feeding of a toxic herring meal (equivalent to 0.1 mg DMN/kg body weight) to 2 cows revealed no detectable harmful effect after 2 years (Koppang, 1970). Of all the animals tested, mink appears to be the most susceptible to the toxic action of DMN. A dietary level of 2.5 or 5 ppm has been reported to produce toxic symptoms within 7–11 days and 100% mortality within 34 days (Carter *et al.*, 1969). Widespread necrosis of the liver accompanied by bile-duct proliferation, ascites, and gastrointestinal hemorrhage were observed in the affected animals.

B. Carcinogenicity

Magee and Barnes (1956) were the first to show that DMN at a level of 50 ppm in the normal diet produced high incidence of malignant liver tumors in rats within 26–40 weeks. At higher dose levels (up to 200 ppm in the food) for a shorter period kidney tumors were observed. Even a single dose of 30 mg/kg body weight produced renal tumors in rats (Magee and Barnes, 1959, 1962). Two different types of renal tumors were observed; one was similar to the renal adenocarcinoma in man, and the other had some resemblance to nephroblastoma. These observations sparked a great deal of interest among scientists and led to the investigation of the carcinogenicity of many other nitrosamines in various species. In this regard, the works by Magee and his co-workers in England, and Druckrey and his associates in Germany deserve special mention for their great contributions to the understanding of the problem.

The remarkable capacity of nitrosamines to induce tumors in different species and different organs is well illustrated from the data presented in Table III. These compounds have been shown to be carcinogenic in 12 species, including monkey. Very few types of compounds are equal to nitrosamines in this respect. As all species of animals so far tested have either succumbed to the carcinogenic action of nitrosamines or died due to extreme toxicity of the compounds it is highly likely that man is also susceptible, although direct evidence of their carcinogenic action in man is lacking. The data presented in Table III are only a few examples, and much more information can be obtained from the review articles mentioned earlier.

The site of action depends to some extent on the structure of the compound and sometimes on the age and species. Druckrey et al. (1967) have examined 65 different nitrosamines, mainly in BD-inbred strain of rats, and attempted to correlate the chemical structure of the compounds to the tumor-bearing organ. The symmetrical dialkylnitrosamines up to diamylnitrosamine, after continuous oral administration to rats, produced liver tumors with decreasing frequency. The only exception was di-n-butylnitrosamine which also produced carcinoma of the urinary bladder. Di-n-amylnitrosamine produced liver and lung tumors; bladder cancer was never observed with this compound (Druckrey and Preussmann, 1962a; Druckrey et al., 1961). The asymmetric dialkylnitrosamines induced tumors of the esophagus (Druckrey et al., 1963a,d; Weisburger et al., 1966). The methyl alkyl nitrosamines were the most active of all, and the effect was completely independent of the route of administration. Methyl allyl nitrosamine was the exception in this group. In addition to the

TABLE III
The Carcinogenic Activity of Some Nitroso Compounds[a]

Compound	Species	Organ	Treatment[b]
DMN	Rat	Liver	Feeding L.S.
		Kidney	Feeding 1–12 wk.
			S.C. and oral 1–10 doses
		Lung	Feeding and daily dosing P.O.
		Nasal sinus	Inhalation, single and repeated
	Mouse	Liver	Feeding L.S.
		Kidney, lung	Drinking L.S. and S.C.
	Hamster	Liver	Drinking water L.S.
	Trout	Liver	Feeding
DEN	Rat	Liver	Drinking L.S.
			Per rectum 5× weekly L.S.
			Single oral
		Kidney	Single oral or I.V.
		Esophagus	Drinking L.S.
	Mouse	Liver	Drinking L.S.
		Stomach and Esophagus	Drinking 30 wk.
		Nose	Percut. daily 6 wk.
	Guinea pig	Liver and Lung	Drinking water 30–40 wk.
	Rabbit	Liver	Drinking water approx. 80 wk.
	Dog	Liver	Food and drinking water
	Monkey	Liver	Daily oral from birth
	Fish	Liver	Water
	Hamster	Liver	Oral 2× weekly, 7 months
			I.P., Percut. intradermal 1× wk.
		Lung and Bronchi	Oral 2× weekly
			I.P., Percut. intradermal 1× wk.
			Transplacental in pregnant hamsters
		Nose	S.C., I.P., intradermal Percut.
Di-*n*-butylnitrosamine	Rat	Liver	Feeding L.S. 75 mg kg⁻¹ day⁻¹
		Bladder and Esophagus	Feeding L.S. 37 mg kg⁻¹ day⁻¹
		Bladder	S.C. 200 mg/kg 1× wk.

Table III (*cont.*)

Compound	Species	Organ	Treatment[b]
n-Butyl-4-hydroxy-butylnitrosamine	Rat	Bladder	Drinking water L.S.
Nitrosopiperidine	Rat	Nose	S.C. 2× wk.
		Esophagus	Drinking water L.S.
		Liver	Drinking water L.S.
	Hamster	Lung	S.C. 2× wk.
Nitrososarcosine	Rat	Esophagus	Drinking water L.S.

[a] A survey of species tested, the organ in which tumors developed, and an outline of the treatment administered. Reproduced from Magee and Barnes (1967), Copyright, Academic Press, Inc.

[b] L.S. = life span; S.C. = subcutaneous injection; I.P. = intraperitoneal injection; Percut. = percutaneous; P.O. = orally.

esophageal cancer it also produced kidney and liver tumors. With the cyclic nitrosamines, however, the site of action was not so specific; some (e.g., nitrosopyrrolidine) affected the liver, while others (nitrosopiperidine, N,N'-dinitrosopiperazine) led to carcinomas of the esophagus. Nitrosamines with functional groups (e.g., compounds with hydroxyl or carboxylic acid groups) were active specifically in the liver, esophagus, or bladder. Several nitrosamines, namely, diallyl-, dicyclohexyl-, diphenyl-, dibenzyl-, *tert*-butylethylnitrosamines as well as trinitrosotrimethylenetriamine, nitrosoindoline, and ethylnitrosoproline displayed no carcinogenic activity.

Recent work by Goodall *et al.* (1968) and Lijinsky *et al.* (1969) has shown that nitroso derivatives of hexamethyleneimine, heptamethyleneimine, and octamethyleneimine also produce cancer of the liver, lungs, or the esophagus. The C-nitroso compound p-nitroso-N,N-dimethylaniline produced a low but significant number of tumors in the esophagus and stomach of rats (Goodall *et al.*, 1968). This appears to be the first occasion where carcinogenesis by a C-nitroso compound has been observed. Some compounds produced tumors in other organs such as the nasal cavity, olfactory nerve, brain, spinal cord, and peripheral nervous system. For example, both nitrosopiperidine and N,N'-dinitrosopiperazine, after subcutaneous injections in rats, produced carcinomas of the ethmoturbinal area and neuroesthesioepitheliomas of the olfactory nerve (Druckrey *et al.*, 1964a). Similar tumors have been observed in golden hamsters after subcutaneous injections of DEN (Herrold, 1964).

The size and frequency of doses are very important in the development of tumors in experimental animals. Scientists believe that a sufficiently low dosage exists below which tumor incidence is statistically indistinguishable from that in control animals. However, a no-effect level for DMN in rats has not been established even after reducing the dietary level of DMN to 2 ppm (Terracini *et al.*, 1967). A single rat on the 2 ppm level of DMN in the diet developed a liver tumor. Druckrey *et al.* (1963c), based on a study of the dose–response relationship with regard to carcinogenesis by DEN in rats, concluded that the carcinogenic effect of DEN increases with time and proposed the following equation:

$$d \times t^{2.3} = \text{constant}$$

where d represents the daily dose, and t the latent period of tumor induction. Even the very low dose of 0.15 mg/kg body weight led to carcinomas in almost all surviving animals (27 out of 30). The average induction time was 609 ± 38 days. With the lowest dose studied, namely 0.075 mg/kg body weight, all four of the surviving rats had liver tumors after 830 days of treatment. This would have been accurately predicted from the above-mentioned equation. A threshold dose was not demonstrable. A study of hemangioendothelioma induced in mice by DEN has shown that on reducing the daily intake of DEN, the total dose necessary to produce tumors also decreases, thus indicating an acceleration process. Schmaehl and Thomas (1965) have also noticed a similar accelerating phenomenon in mice. In another study, Arcos *et al.* (1969) concluded that, under the experimental conditions used, the minimum total effective tumor dose of DEN in guinea pigs was 86 mg. Multiple liver tumors have been produced in mink after prolonged feeding of 0.05 mg DMN kg⁻¹ body weight day⁻¹ (Koppang, 1970). The liver tumors in such cases seldom metastasized; the most common type observed was the hemangiomas which was prone to rupture and cause death due to bleeding.

One of the remarkable features of the nitroso compounds is their capacity to cause cancer in the progeny of animals treated during pregnancy. Mohr *et al.* (1965, 1966) administered DEN to pregnant hamsters and observed tracheal papillomas and liver damage in the 25-week-old young offsprings. It was also established that the young of untreated mothers, when suckled by treated mothers, did not show any pathological symptoms, thus eliminating the possibility of transfer of DEN via the milk (Mohr and Althoff, 1965). Similarly, Alexandrov (1968) was able to induce renal tumors in the offspring of rats after administration of DMN during the gestation period. Transplacental carcinogenesis in rats has also been reported after administration of several other nitrosamines such as methyl- and ethylnitrosoaniline (Napalkov and Alexandrov, 1968). Thomas and Bollmann (1968), however, noticed only weak transplacental carcinogenic effects in Wistar rats given DEN during pregnancy. No evidence for a teratogenic effect due to the administration of dialkylnitrosamines has so far been reported (Thomas and Bollmann, 1968; Napalkov and Alexandrov, 1968).

C. FACTORS AFFECTING TUMOR PRODUCTION

Age is an important factor affecting the carcinogenic response of an animal to nitrosamines. For example, DMN induced tumors in the liver, kidney, and lung in adult Swiss mice but only produced liver and lung tumors in the newborn (Terracini *et al.,* 1966). Kidneys of newborn mice were highly resistant to the carcinogenic action of DMN. This was believed to be due to their inability to metabolize DMN and produce the necessary proximate carcinogen (Section VI, E). Toth *et al.* (1964), on the other hand, have observed liver carcinomas in newborn mice but not in the adults after treatment with DMN. There is also an increased tumor incidence with a shorter latent period in the young animals (H. C. Grice, personal communication).

Sex may also have some effect on the carcinogenic response, but very little information is available at the moment. Lee and Goodall (1968) reported the induction of tumors in hypophysectomized rats after treatment with DMN. This is in contrast to the well-known inhibitory action of this technique on tumor induction by other carcinogens such as azo dyes, acetylaminofluorene, and aflatoxin. A report by Reuber and Lee (1968) indicates that both age and sex are important factors in the hepatocarcinogenic response to DEN in Buffalo rats. These workers showed that the incidence of liver tumors was greater in animals in which the treatment was initiated at an early age and became progressively less frequent as the starting age increased. Moreover, the younger females had a higher incidence of liver carcinoma than the males of the same age group, and none of the females developed cirrhosis of the liver. Vesselinovitch (1969) also observed higher incidence of liver tumors in male mice than in females after treatment with DMN early in life (7 days old).

The nutritional status of animals has been reported to be another factor affecting carcinogenesis by nitrosamines. Thus, Swann and McLean (1968) observed that rats maintained on a protein-free diet were more likely to have kidney tumors after treatment with DMN. It was demonstrated that the metabolism of DMN by the liver, but not by the kidney, was reduced considerably. Under such conditions, most of the DMN was metabolized by the kidney (hence produced the proximate carcinogen), thus explaining the increased incidence of kidney tumors in the experimental animals. Khanna and Puri (1966) studied the effect of diets rich or deficient in protein, cystine, and choline on the toxic effect of DMN in rats. An enriched diet considerably reduced the hepatic damage and also helped to overcome the damage much quicker, while the deficient diet had exactly the opposite effects. Lacassagne et al. (1967) and Osswald and Schmaehl (1966) failed to observe any clear-cut influence of diets on the hepatocarcinogenic effect by DEN in rats.

The toxic and carcinogenic activity of nitrosamines can also be influenced by other chemicals. Montesano and Saffiotti (1968) have shown that simultaneous administration of DEN and a polycyclic hydrocarbon greatly increased the incidence of respiratory tumors.

Either of these chemicals, when given singly, produced only a few, if any, tumors at the dose used. These workers also demonstrated that intratracheal instillation of ferric oxide particles can have a synergistic action on the carcinogenesis by DEN, 3-Methylcholanthrene and other polynuclear aromatic hydrocarbons are known to induce *de novo* synthesis of N-demethylase enzymes in hepatic and nonhepatic tissues. It was thought, therefore, that simultaneous administration of 3-methylcholanthrene and DMN would enhance carcinogenicity of DMN. But, surprisingly enough, Venkatesan *et al.* (1968) observed that such treatments decreased the incidence of liver tumors in rats but at the same time increased the occurrence of lung tumors. No lung tumor was noticed in the control rats that received either DMN or 3-methylcholanthrene. The presence of a microsomal mixed-function oxidase enzyme system in the rat liver was described that catalyzed the oxidative demethylation of DMN. It was later concluded (Venkatesan *et al.*, 1970a) that the inhibitory effect of 3-methylcholanthrene was due to the inhibition in the synthesis of the DMN-demethylase enzyme.

The activity of the above-mentioned enzyme was markedly enhanced in fasted rats. The ingestion of glucose alone had an inhibitory effect on the activity of DMN-demethylase, whereas that of casein had the reverse effect (Venkatesan *et al.*, 1970b). McLean and Magee (1970) have shown that rats on a protein-deficient diet are protected against the acute toxic effect of DMN but are more prone to the late carcinogenic action of the compound. Phenobarbitone and DDT had no protective effect against the carcinogenic action of DMN on the kidney.

Phenobarbitone was found to increase the total dose of DEN required to cause death by tumor induction in mice (Kunz *et al.*, 1969). It also reduced the number of malignant tumors in the liver but significantly increased carcinomas of the stomach. Halothane and methoxyflurane did not have any noticeable effect on the survival time, tumor frequency, and tumor localization in mice treated with DEN. It is interesting to note, however, that each of these enzyme inducers altered the ratio of hemangioendotheliomas to liver cancers induced in the liver by DEN. Reserpine has also been reported to reduce the hepatocarcinogenicity of DEN in rats (Lacassagne *et al.*, 1968).

D. MUTAGENESIS

Various nitrosamines and nitrosamides are mutagenic to the fruit fly *Drosophila* (Pasternak, 1964). As in the case of transplacental carcinogenesis the nitrosamides are much more active mutagens than the nitrosamines. The nitrosamines are mutagenic only in *Drosophila* and in the plant *Arabidopsis thaliana* (Veleminsky and Gichner, 1968), but not in the microorganisms such as *E. coli, Neurospora,* and *Saccharomyces.* The nitrosamides are mutagenic in most of these organisms (Marquardt *et al.,* 1963a,b, 1964; Geissler, 1962; Trams and Kuenkel, 1964). This difference in activity between the nitrosamines and nitrosamides may be explained by the fact that the latter type of compounds are unstable, and they spontaneously break down to the active agents, whereas the former group of compounds require metabolic activation before imparting their biological actions (Section VI,E). However, there are still some unexplained facts which are not consistent with this hypothesis, and further work is needed to fully understand the mutagenic process (Fahmy *et al.,* 1966; Loveless, 1969).

E. METABOLISM AND MODE OF ACTION

Magee (1956) studied the metabolism of DMN in rats, mice, and rabbits and reported that it was metabolized very rapidly, and that metabolism was nearly complete within 24 hours. Very little unchanged DMN was excreted in the feces or urine. Most of the metabolism took place in the liver, although lower rates of metabolism in other organs could not be excluded. Later studies (Dutton and Heath, 1956) with C^{14}-labeled DMN established that about 65% of the injected C^{14} could be recovered in the expired carbon dioxide within 6 hours of a subcutaneous dose (50 mg/kg body weight) to mice. The metabolism in the rat was a little slower. The rest of the radioactivity was evenly distributed in the tissues, and some (about 7%) was excreted in the urine. Magee and Vandekar (1958) also studied the metabolic breakdown of DMN *in vitro,* using tissue slices or homogenates, and followed the disappearance of DMN. The reaction rate was fastest in the presence of oxygen and slower in the presence of air. No detectable decomposition took place in nitrogen atmosphere. Among the organs tested liver was the most active, and all other organs (except the kidney) such as spleen, heart, and lung did not metabolize the nitrosamines. *In vitro* experiments with rat liver microsome preparations established that formaldehyde was one of the metabolic products of DMN (Brouwers and Emmelot, 1960), and DEN was converted to acetaldehyde by a similar oxidative dealkylation process (Mizrahi and Emmelot, 1962).

It was clear from the work of Heath (1962) that the dialkylnitrosamines themselves were not responsible for their toxic actions because any treatment which increased their persistence *in vivo* failed to increase the toxicity of the compounds. The suggestion that diazoalkanes may be produced from the nitrosamines to act as the proximate carcinogen led Heath (1961) to compare the toxic properties of several alkylnitrosamines. As expected, methyl-*n*-butylnitrosamine, which can undergo α-oxidation to form diazomethane or diazobutane, caused acute centrilobular necrosis in rats, but the corresponding isomer *tert*-butylmethylnitrosamine did not cause the typical necrosis of the liver even after high doses for a period of 4 consecutive days. On chemical grounds, the metabolism of *tert*-butylmethylnitrosamine can not yield a diazoalkane and, therefore, the results were in good agreement with this theory. The identification of 7-methylguanine in the nucleic acids isolated from the liver of rats treated with DMN also gave support to the theory that an alkylating agent, either diazomethane or a carbonium ion, is formed from DMN (Magee and Hultin, 1962; Magee and Farber, 1962). The methylation of guanine in both RNA and DNA fractions of the liver was observed. Craddock and Magee (1963) later presented evidence for the methylation of DNA of kidney and isolated 7-methylguanine in acid hydrolysates of the nucleic acid obtained from this organ of rats treated with radioactive DMN. These workers also studied the extent and rate of methylation of RNA and DNA in rats and mice (Craddock and Magee 1963, 1965). More recently, Montesano and Magee (1970) have studied the metabolism of C^{14}-DMN in human liver slices by measuring the production of radioactive carbon dioxide. The rate of carbon dioxide production and the amount of 7-

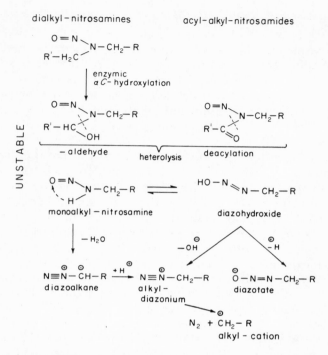

Fig. 3. Proposed mechanism for the formation of alkylating intermediates from dialkylnitrosamines and acylalkylnitrosamides. (Taken from Druckrey *et al.*, 1969. With permission of the New York Academy of Sciences.)

methylguanine in the nucleic acid formed in the reaction mixture were comparable to that obtained with rat liver slices. In view of these results it was concluded that man is probably as sensitive as the rat to the carcinogenic action of DMN.

It has become clear from various studies that the first step in the activation of DMN is the oxidative dealkylation process leading to the formation of formaldehyde and monomethylnitrosamine which decomposes spontaneously, due to its extreme instability, to yield diazomethane or methylene or methyl carbonium ion. For biochemical reasons, however, Druckrey *et al.* (1961) thought that the first step of activation is an enzymic hydroxylation on an αC

atom. The αC-hydroxyalkylnitrosamine then dealkylates spontaneously to the monoalkylnitrosamine which by protonic change forms the isomeric diazohydroxide as depicted in Fig. 3. The subsequent intermediates, namely, diazoalkane, diazotate, or alkyldiazonium compounds can be formed as shown in the diagram. The alkyldiazonium compound is highly reactive; it can lead to diazotization or can decompose to the alkylcarbonium ion which is probably the proximate carcinogen. The mechanism of action of cycasin, a naturally occurring toxin present in cycads, and its aglycone methylazoxymethanol is believed to be similar to that of DMN (Miller, 1964). The acylalkylnitrosamides undergo spontaneous heterolysis, and the further degradative pathways are the same as in the case of the nitrosamines. The theory fits in very well with the observed lack of carcinogenicity of *tert*-butylethylnitrosamine (Druckrey *et al.*, 1963a). The *tert*-butyl group lacks an αC atom, and, therefore, cannot be oxidized to produce the diazoalkane (Fig. 1). Among all the steps described in Fig. 3 only the initial αC-hydroxylation process is enzymic, and it is probably responsible for the organotropic effects which have been observed with the liver carcinogen, DMN (Magee and Barnes, 1956). It is noteworthy that di-n-butylnitrosamine is the only symmetrical dialkylnitrosamine which produces bladder cancer in rats (Section VI,B), and it is believed that n-butyl-4-hydroxybutylnitrosamine or its conjugates, which can be formed from the parent nitrosamine by hydroxylation of an alkyl group, are the actual bladder carcinogens (Druckrey *et al.*, 1964b). This hydroxylation process probably takes place in the bladder mucosa.

Recently Lijinsky *et al.* (1968) applied mass spectrometric technique to study the mechanism of methylation of nucleic acids in rats with deuterated DMN. These workers concluded that the predominant alkylating agent is the carbonium ion and not diazomethane. Although the amount of 7-methylguanine formed in various organs has been frequently correlated with the susceptibility of that organ to the carcinogenic action of an individual nitrosamine, there are many discrepancies that cannot be explained (Magee and Barnes, 1967; Lijinsky and Ross, 1969). The results obtained so far indicate, however, that at least in the case of some

nitrosamines the alkylation process of nucleic acids plays an important role in mutagenesis and carcinogenesis.

F. BIOCHEMICAL EFFECTS

One of the early biochemical effects reported to occur after injection of a necrotizing dose of DMN is impairment of amino acid
incorporation into liver proteins (Magee, 1958; Brouwers and
Emmelot, 1960; Hultin *et al.,* 1960). Biochemical studies with intact
animals and in isolated microsome plus cell-sap isolates suggested
that the initial damage may have occurred in the microsome struc-
tures. The inhibitory effect of DMN on the synthesis of hepatic
proteins was shown to be quite specific as it did not affect other
enzymic activities (Brouwers and Emmelot, 1960). Emmelot and
Benedetti (1960, 1961) reported progressive loss of glycogen from
livers of DMN-treated rats. However, this loss of glycogen was
not visible within the first 3 hours of the treatment. It was also
observed that subcutaneous injection of cysteine reduced the
inhibitory action of DMN on protein synthesis and the loss of
glycogen, but apparently had no such protective action against DEN
(Emmelot and Mizrahi, 1961; Emmelot *et al.,* 1962; Mizrahi and
Emmelot, 1962, 1963). Cysteamine, on the other hand, exerted
a protective effect on the inhibition of hepatic protein synthesis
in animals treated with DMN or DEN. It was concluded that the
protective effect of cysteine and cysteamine may have been man-
ifested either by competitive reaction with the diazoalkanes formed
in situ from the nitrosamines, or by inhibiting the initial breakdown
of the nitrosamines by the dealkylating enzymes.

While studying the effect of DMN in sheep Sakshaug *et al.* (1965)
observed an increase in the plasma glutamic transaminase and
ornithine carbamyl transferase activities after varying doses (0.25–5
mg/kg body weight) of the test compound. These changes were
observed 1–6 days before any clinical symptoms appeared. The
plasma glutamic pyruvic transaminase activity was normal in most
cases with the exception of two sheep in which a moderate increase
was seen just before death occurred. Hyperbilirubinemia was
observed in a few cases. The effects of nitrosamines on the levels

of other enzymes have been discussed in the review articles mentioned earlier.

VII. Other *N*-Nitroso Compounds

These include various types of nitrosoureas, nitroso guanidines, and nitrosamino acids. Brief mention has already been made about these compounds throughout this text. As far as the author is aware there is no published report of the occurrence of these chemicals in foods. The main difficulty has been the lack of sufficiently sensitive analytical methods. Furthermore, the nitrosoureas are very unstable in aqueous solution, and they react easily with sulfhydryl groups (Section II,D). Therefore, these compounds, if present or formed in foods, will be very short-lived. However, the danger of their formation in the stomach from nitrite and the amide components and subsequent manifestation of their carcinogenic property is a real possibility. This has already been demonstrated to happen in experimental animals (Section III,D).

Nitrosoureas and nitrosoguanidines have been shown to induce tumors in the stomach, esophagus, lung, kidney, intestine, brain, skin, and spinal cord. The nitrosoureas and nitrosoguanidines are also strong mutagenic agents. Some of the nitrosourea compounds are strong teratogens as well as transplacental carcinogens (Sections III,D and VI,B,D). A current review of the literature concerning the carcinogenicity of various nitrosoureas and nitrosoguanidines has been published (BIBRA Bull., 1971).

Among this group of compounds the nitrosamino acids and their metabolites are the most likely ones to be encountered in foods. Nitrososarcosine, nitrosoproline, and nitrosocitrulline all can be derived from the corresponding amino compounds (Section III,C). Nitrosomethylurea can be formed from nitrite and methylguanidine which occurs in beef and fish (Section III,C). It might be worthwhile to mention that a naturally occurring compound streptozotocin, an antibiotic produced by *Streptomyces achromogenes,* is a substituted nitrosourea compound (Herr *et al.,* 1967), and it has been shown to induce kidney tumors in the rat (Arison and

Feudale, 1967). As these fungi are widespread in nature the possibility that they may contaminate human foods cannot be dismissed. Further research may reveal the existence of other new nitroso compounds which could be present in foods or formed in the stomach from their precursors.

VIII. Possible Human Health Hazards

From the foregoing discussion there can be little doubt that nitrosamines and other related nitroso compounds are powerful carcinogens, and their presence in foods or the environment constitutes a potential health hazard to humans. The available evidence indicates that only trace amounts of nitrosamines, mainly DMN and DEN, are present in isolated samples of some foods, especially those preserved with nitrate or nitrite. However, these data were obtained from the analysis of only a limited number of samples which can hardly be considered as representative of all the foods consumed by man in different countries. Further surveys of a wider range of products are needed before an estimation of the average daily intake of nitrosamines by humans can be made. Moreover, some of the results reported in the literature may be unreliable because nonspecific methods were used in the analysis.

The possibility of the formation of various nitroso compounds from their precursors in the stomach may represent a greater threat to human health than could be anticipated from the low natural levels present in foods. However, at present there is not sufficient information available concerning the amount and nature of various nitrosatable amino compounds in foods to assess the extent of the hazard that exists to man.

The question arises whether there is an "acceptable" or "tolerable" level of nitrosamines in foods for human consumption. For evaluating the safety of a food additive or contaminant it is customary to use a 100-fold safety factor over the no-effect level observed in animal experiments. As mentioned earlier (Section VI,B), Terracini *et al.* (1967) have failed to find such a no-effect level of DMN in rats. A concentration of 2 ppm DMN in the diet was carcinogenic. A daily dose of 0.05 mg DMN/kg body weight, which is equivalent to approximately 0.2–0.5 ppm in the diet, has also produced liver tumors in minks (Section VI,B). Similar studies by Druckrey *et al.* (1963c) have established that DEN is equally effective in producing cancer in rats at low doses. Therefore, a "threshold" concentration of DMN or DEN in experimental animals has not been established. In the absence of reliable data on dose–response relationships at low levels it is difficult to assess the hazard to human health arising from exposures to trace amounts of nitrosamines. In view of the extreme carcinogenicity of the nitrosamines and their capacity to induce cancer in the offspring it is highly desirable to have foods free of these compounds. In practice, however, it is not always possible to reach this goal, and trace amounts of nitrosamines are bound to be encountered in some samples. Efforts should, therefore, be made to keep the level of nitrosamines in foods as low as possible and preferably below the level of 5 ppb. It is hoped that further research on the origin of various amines and nitrosamines and the development of better techniques of food preservation will greatly facilitate the achievement of this goal.

IX. Areas of Future Research

Despite the excellent progress made during recent years in the research on nitrosamines in foods there are still some gaps in our understanding of the problem. The major and most urgent issue seems to be our lack of knowledge of the nonvolatile nitrosamines and related compounds such as nitrosamino acids, nitrosoureas, and nitrosoguanidines. Much more effort should be made in exploring these areas. A general screening method for all *N*-nitroso compounds will be useful. Research should also be carried out to determine the levels of various *N*-nitrosatable organic compounds in foods. Since the naturally occurring amino compounds are always likely to be present in foods, the chance of their conversion to the corresponding nitroso derivatives can be greatly minimized by reducing the levels of nitrite in the diet.

The first step may be to find an alternative preserving agent that can replace nitrate or nitrite in meat, fish, and cheese without minimizing the protection these chemicals offer against *Clostridium* poisoning. Another area of research that has been so far neglected is the role of foodborne microorganisms in the synthesis of nitrosamines. As fish, meat, and cheese contain many amines and some of these foods also contain added nitrate or nitrite, there is a real possibility that certain microorganisms do contribute to some extent to the formation of nitrosamines in these products.

Experimental work with laboratory animals suggests that tumors produced by N-nitroso compounds in some cases are similar in appearance to those found in man. The nitrosamines are carcinogenic in a wide range of organs, and some of them are highly organ-specific. It is not unreasonable to suggest that there may be some relation between the occurrence of nitrosamines in the environment and human cancer. Careful epidemiological studies will be necessary to establish such a relationship. Such studies should be encouraged especially in areas where a particular type of cancer is more prevalent than that found in other parts of the world. However, it should be strongly emphasized that this is only a possibility, and at present there is no evidence to suggest that nitrosamines in the environment or foods are partly responsible for human cancer. Major research programs in the areas mentioned above are urgently needed to fill in the gaps in our knowledge of nitrosamines in foods and their possible relationship in the etiology of human cancer.

References*

Alam, B.S., Saporoschetz, I. B., and Epstein, S. S. (1971a). *Nature (London)* **232,** 116.
Alam, B.S., Saporoschetz, I. B., and Epstein, S. S. (1971b). *Nature (London)* **232,** 199.
Alexandrov, V. A. (1968). *Nature (London)* **218,** 280.
Althorpe, J., Goddard, D. A., Sissons, D. J., and Telling, G. M. (1970). *J. Chromatgr.* **53,** 371.

*References marked with asterisk are to papers presented at the meeting of the International Agency for Research on Cancer (IARC), Lyon, and Deutsches Krebsforschungszentrum, Heidelberg, which was held October 13–15, 1971, in Heidelberg. The topic of the meeting was "Analysis and Formation of Nitrosamines." The proceedings will be published by IARC in their monograph series.

Amano, K., and Tozawa, H. (1965). *In* "Freezing and Irradiation of Fish" (R. Kreuzer, ed.), pp. 467–471. Fishing News (Books) Ltd., London.

Anonymous (1969). *Food Cosmet. Toxicol.* **7**, 243.

Arcos, J. C., Argus, M. F., and Matheson, J. B. (1969). *Experientia* **25**, 296.

Arison, R. N., and Feudale, E. L. (1967). *Nature (London)* **214**, 1254.

Barnes, J. M., and Magee, P. N. (1954). *Brit. J. Ind. Med.* **11**, 167.

Beatty, S. A., and Gibbons, N. E. (1937). *J. Biol. Bd. Can.* **3**, 77.

Bodansky, C. (1951). *Pharmacol. Rev.* **3**, 144.

Bogovski, P., Castegnaro, M., Pignatelli, B., and Walker, E. A. (1971). The retardation effect of tannins on the formation of nitrosamines.*

Bøhler, N. (1960). *Nor. Pelsdyrbl.* **34**, 104.

Bøhler, N. (1962). *Nord. Veterinaermoede, Beretn., 9th,* 1962. Vol. 2, p. 774.

Borgstrom, G., ed. (1961). "Fish as Food," Vol. 1. Academic Press, New York.

Boyland, E., Nice, E., and Williams, K. (1971). *Food Cosmet. Toxicol.* **9**, 1.

British Industries. (1971). *Biol. Res. Ass. Bull.* **3**, 117.

Brouwers, J. A. J., and Emmelot, P. (1960). *Exp. Cell Res.* **19**, 467.

Budzikiewicz, H., Djerassi, C., and Williams, D.H. (1967). "Mass Spectrometry of Organic Compounds," pp. 329 and 523. Holden-Day, San Francisco, California.

Burks, R. E., Baker, E. B., Clark, P., Esslinger, J., and Lacey, J. C. (1959). *J. Agr. Food Chem.* **7**, 778.

Canadian Food and Drug Act and Regulations. (1965). Table XI. Queen's Printer and Controller of Stationery, Ottawa.

Cantoni, C., Bianchi, M. A., Rennon, P., and D'Aubert, S. (1969). *Arch. Vet. Ital.* **20**, 245.

Carlton, W. W., and Wesler, J. R. (1968). *Toxicol. Appl. Pharmacol.* **13**, 404.

Carter, R. L., Percival, W. H., and Roe, F. J. C. (1969). *J. Pathol.* **97**, 79.

Castell, C. H., Neal, W., and Smith, B. (1970). *J. Fish. Res. Bd. Can.* **27**, 1685.

Castell, C. H., Smith, B., and Neal, W. (1971). *J. Fish. Res. Bd. Can.* **28**, 1.

Chemical Rubber Company (1966–1967). The Handbook of Chemistry and Physics, 47th Ed. The Chemical Rubber Company, Cleveland, Ohio.

Chow, Y. L. (1967). *Can. J. Chem.* **45**, 53.

Collin, J. (1954). *Bull. Soc. Roy. Sci. Liege* **23**, 201.

Courts, A. (1970). *Nature (London)* **225**, 302.

Craddock, V. M., and Magee, P. N. (1963). *Biochem. J.* **89**, 32.

Craddock, V. M., and Magee, P. N. (1965). *Biochim. Biophys. Acta* **95**, 677.

Crosby, N. T., Foreman, J. K., and Palframan, J. F. (1971).*

Daiber, D., and Preussmann, R. (1964). *Z. Anal. Chem.* **206**, 344.

Dehove, R. A. (1970). *In* "La réglementation des produits alimentaires et non alimentaires," 7th ed., p. 200. Commerce Editions, Paris.

Devik, O. G. (1967). *Acta Chem. Scand.* **21**, 2302.

Druckrey, H., and Preussmann, R. (1962a). *Naturwissenschaften* **49**, 111.

Druckrey, H., and Preussmann, R. (1962b). *Naturwissenschaften* **49**, 498.

Druckrey, H., Preussmann, R., Schmaehl, D., and Mueller, M. (1961). *Naturwissenschaften* **48**, 134.

Druckrey, H., Preussmann, R., Blum, G., Ivankovic, S., and Afkham, J. (1963a). *Naturwissenschaften* **50,** 100.

Druckrey, H., Steinhoff, D., and Beuthner, H. (1963b). *Arzneim-Forsch.* **13,** 320.

Druckrey, H., Schildbach, A., Schmaehl, D., Preussmann, R., and Ivankovic, S. (1963c). *Arzneim-Forsch.* **13,** 841.

Druckrey, H., Preussmann, R., and Schmaehl, D. (1963d). *Acta Unio Int. Contra Cancrum* **19,** 510.

Druckrey, H., Ivankovic, S., Mennel, H. D., and Preussmann, R. (1964a). *Z. Krebsforsch.* **66,** 138.

Druckrey, H., Preussmann, R., Ivankovic, S., Schmidt, C. H., Mennel, H. D., and Stahl, K. W. (1964b). *Z. Krebsforsch.* **66,** 280.

Druckrey, H., Preussmann, R., Ivankovic, S., and Schmaehl, D. (1967). *Z. Krebsforsch.* **69,** 103.

Druckrey, H., Preussmann, R., and Ivankovic, S. (1969). *Ann. N. Y. Acad. Sci.* **163,** 676–696.

Dubrow, H., and Kabisch, W. (1960). *Milchwissenschaft* **15,** 543.

DuPlessis, L. S., Nunn, J. R., and Roach, W. A. (1969). *Nature (London)* **222,** 1198.

Dutton, A. H., and Heath, D. F. (1956). *Nature (London)* **178,** 644.

Eddy, B. P., and Ingram, M. (1962). *Food Sci. Technol. Proc. Int. Cong., 1st, 1962* **2,** 405.

Eisenbrand, G. (1971). * Unpublished paper.

Eisenbrand, G., and Preussmann, R. (1970). *Arzneim.-Forsch.* **20,** 3.

Eisenbrand, G., Marquardt, P., and Preussmann, R. (1969). *Z. Anal. Chem.* **247,** 54.

Eisenbrand, G., Hodenberg, A. V., and Preussmann, R. (1970a). *Z. Anal. Chem.* **251,** 22.

Eisenbrand, G., Spaczynski, K., and Preussmann, R. (1970b). *J. Chromatogr.* **51,** 304.

Eisenbrand, G., Spaczynski, K., and Preussmann, R. (1970c). *J. Chromatogr.* **51,** 503.

Emmelot, P., and Benedetti, E. L. (1960). *J. Biophys. Biochem. Cytol.* **7,** 393.

Emmelot, P., and Benedetti, E. L. (1961). *In* "Protein Biosynthesis" (R. J. C. Harris, ed.), pp. 99–123. Academic Press, New York.

Emmelot, P., and Mizrahi, I. J. (1961). *Nature (London)* **192,** 42.

Emmelot, P., Mizrahi, I. J., and Kriek, E. (1962). *Nature (London)* **193,** 1158.

Emmons, W. D. (1954). *J. Amer. Chem. Soc.* **76,** 3468.

Ender, F. (1966). *Int. Tag. Weltges. Buiatrik, 4th, 1966* p. 1.

Ender, F., and Ceh, L. (1967). *Alkylierend Wirkende Verbindungen, Conf. Tobacco Res. 2nd, 1960,* p. 83.

Ender, F., and Ceh, L. (1971). *Z. Lebensm.-Unters.-Forsch.* **145,** 133.

Ender, F., Havre, G., Helgebostad, A., Koppang, N., Madsen, R., and Ceh, L. (1964). *Naturwissenschaften* **51,** 637.

Ender, F., Havre, G. N., Madsen, R., Ceh, L., and Helgebostad, A. (1967). *Z. Tierphysiol., Tierernaehr. Futtermittelk.* **22,** 181.

Fahmy, O. G., Fahmy, M. J., Massasso, J., and Ondrej, M. (1966). *Mutat. Res.* **3,** 201.

Fassett, D. W. (1966). *Nat. Acad. Sci.–Nat. Res. Counc., Publ.* **1354,** 250–256.

Fazio, T., Damico, J. N., Howard, J. W., White, R. H., and Watts, J. O. (1971a). *J. Agr. Food Chem.* **19,** 250.

Fazio, T., White, R. H., and Howard, J. W. (1971b). *J. Ass. Offic. Anal. Chem.* **54,** 1157.

Fazio, T., Howard, J. W., and White, R. (1971c).*

Fiddler, W., Doerr, R. C., Ertel, J. R., and Wasserman, A. E. (1971). *J. Ass. Offic. Anal. Chem.* **54,** 1160.

Fiegl, F. (1955). *Anal. Chem.* **27,** 1315.

Fieser, L. F., and Fieser, M. (1967). "Reagents for Organic Synthesis," pp. 747–749, Wiley, New York.

Fieser, L. F., and Fieser, M. (1968). *In* "Advanced Organic Chemistry," pp. 377, 508, and 717–718. Van Nostrand-Reinhold, Princeton, New Jersey.

Fong, Y. Y., and Walsh, E. O'F. (1971). *Lancet* **2,** 1032.

Foreman, J. K., Palframan, J. F., and Walker, E. A. (1970). *Nature (London)* **225,** 554.

Freimuth, U., and Glaeser, E. (1970). *Nahrung* **14,** 357.

Galesloot, T. E. (1956). *Proc. Int. Dairy Congr., 14th, 1956* Part 2, p. 849; *Chem. Abstr.* **51,** 15030a (1957).

Galesloot, T. E. (1964). *Neth. Milk Dairy J.* **18,** 127.

Geissler, E. (1962). *Naturwissenschaften* **49,** 380.

Gerritsen, G. A., and De Willigen, A. H. A. (1969). *Staerke* **21,** 101.

Golovnya, R. V., Zhuravleva, I. L., Mironov, G. A., and Abdullina, R. M. (1970). *Moloch. Prom.* **31,** 8; cited from *Food Sci. Technol. Abstr.* **2,** 8P1024 (1970).

Goodall, C. M., Lijinsky, W., and Tomatis, L. (1968). *Cancer Res.* **28,** 1217.

Greenberg, R. A., and Silliker, J. H. (1961). *J. Food Sci.* **26,** 622.

Greenblatt, M., Mirvish, S., and So, B. T. (1971). *J. Nat. Cancer Inst.* **46,** 1029.

Hartmann, W. W., and Roll, L. J. (1943). *In* "Organic Synthesis, Collective Volume II" (A. H. Blatt, ed.), p. 460. Wiley, New York.

Hatt, H. H. (1943). *In* "Organic Synthesis, Collective Volume II" (A. H. Blatt, ed.), pp. 211–213. Wiley, New York.

Hawksworth, G., and Hill, M. J. (1971). *Biochem. J.* **122,** 28P.

Heath, D. F. (1961). *Nature (London)* **192,** 170.

Heath, D. F. (1962). *Biochem. J.* **85,** 72.

Heath, D. F., and Jarvis, J. A. E. (1955). *Analyst* **80,** 613.

Hedler, L., and Marquardt, P. (1968). *Food Cosmet. Toxicol.* **6,** 341.

Hedler, L., Kaunitz, H., Marquardt, P., Fales, H., and Johnson, R. E. (1971.)*

Hein, G. E. (1963). *J. Chem. Educ.* **40,** 181.

Herr, R. R., Jahnke, H. K., and Argoudelis, A. D. (1967). *J. Amer. Chem. Soc.* **89,** 4808.

Herrmann, H. (1961). *Hoppe-Seyler's Z. Physiol. Chem.* **326,** 13.

Herrmann, H., Jungstand, W., and Schnabel, R. (1966). *Arzneim.-Forsch,* **16,** 1244.

Herrold, K. M. D. (1964). *Cancer* **17,** 114.

Heyns, K., and Koch, H. (1970). *Tetrahedron Lett.* No. 10, p. 741.

Heyns, K., and Roeper, H. (1970). *Tetrahedron Lett.* No. 10, p. 737.

Hill, M. J., and Hawksworth, G. (1971).*

Howard, J. W., Fazio, T., and Watts, J. O. (1970). *J. Ass. Offic. Anal. Chem.* **53,** 269.

Hultin, T., Arrhenius, E., Loew, H., and Magee, P. N. (1960). *Biochem. J.* **76,** 109.

Ingram, M. (1959). *Chem. Ind. (London)* p. 552.

Ingram, M., and Dainty, R. H. (1971). *J. Appl. Bacteriol.* **34,** 21.

Issenberg, P., and Tannenbaum, S. R. (1971). *

Ivankovic, S., and Preussmann, R. (1970). *Naturwissenschaften* **57,** 460.

Ivankovic, S., Druckrey, H., and Preussmann, R. (1965). *Z. Krebsforsch.* **66,** 541.

Kamm, L., McKeown, G. G., and Smith, D. M. (1965). *J. Ass. Offic. Agr. Chem.* **48,** 892

Kapeller-Adler, R., and Krael, J. (1930a). *Biochem. Z.* **221,** 437.

Kapeller-Adler, R., and Krael, J. (1930b). *Biochem. Z.* **224,** 364.

Keybets, J. H., Groot, E. H., and Keller, G. H. M. (1970). *Food Cosmet. Toxicol.* **8,** 167.

Khanna, S. D., and Puri, D. (1966). *J. Pathol. Bacteriol.* **91,** 605.

Kilgore, L., Stasch, A. R., and Barrentine, B. F. (1963). *J. Amer. Diet. Ass.* **43,** 39.

Klubes, P., and Jondroff, W. R. (1971). *Res. Commun. Chem. Pathol. Pharmacol.* **2,** 24.

Komarow, S. A. (1929). *Biochem. Z.* **211,** 326.

Koppang, N. (1964). *Nord. Veterinaermed.* **16,** 305.

Koppang, N. (1970). *Acta Pathol. Microbiol. Scand., Sect. A and B, Suppl.* **215,** 30.

Koppang, N., and Helgebostad, A. (1966). *Nord. Veterinaermed.* **18,** 216.

Kroeller, E. (1967). *Deut. Lebensm.-Rundsch.* **63,** 303.

Kunz, W., Schaude, G., and Thomas, C. (1969). *Z. Krebsforsch.* **72,** 291.

Lacassagne, A., Buu-Hoi, N. P., and Giao, N. B. (1967). *Int. J. Cancer* **2,** 425.

Lacassagne, A., Buu-Hoi, N. P., and Giao, N. B. (1968). *Bull. Cancer* **55,** 87.

Landmann, W. A., and Batzer, O. F. (1966). *J. Agr. Food Chem.* **14,** 210.

Lee, C. Y., Shallenberger, R. S., Downing, D. L., Stoewsand, G. S., and Peck, N. M. (1971). *J. Sci. Food Agr.* **22,** 90.

Lee, K. Y., and Goodall, C. M. (1968). *Biochem. J.* **106,** 767.

Lembke, A., and Moebus, O. (1970). *Proc. Int. Dairy Congr. 18th, 1970* A. 2. 3, p. 29.

Levin, I. W., Milne, G. W. A., and Axenrod, T. (1970). *J. Chem. Phys.* **53,** 2505.

Liener, I. E., ed. (1969). "Toxic Constituents of Plant Foodstuffs." Academic Press, New York.

Lijinsky, W., and Epstein, S. S. (1970). *Nature (London)* **225,** 21.

Lijinsky, W., and Ross, A. E. (1969). *J. Nat. Cancer Inst.* **42,** 1095.

Lijinsky, W., Loo, J., and Ross, A. E. (1968). *Nature (London)* **218,** 1174.

Lijinsky, W., Tomatis, L., and Wenyon, C. E. M. (1969). *Proc. Soc. Exp. Biol. Med.* **130,** 945.

Lijinsky, W., Keefer, L., and Loo, J. (1970). *Tetrahedron* **26,** 5137.

Lintzel, W., Pfeiffer, H., and Zippel, I. (1939). *Biochem. Z.* **301,** 29.

Loveless, A. (1969). *Nature (London)* **233,** 206.

McGlashan, N. D., and Walters, C. L. (1969). *S. Afr. Med. J.* **43,** 800.

McGlashan, N. D., Walters, C. L., and McLean, A. E. M. (1968). *Lancet* **2,** 1017.

McGlashan, N. D., Patterson, R. L. S., and Williams, A. A. (1970). *Lancet* **2,** 1138.

McIlwain, P. K., and Schipper, I. A. (1963). *J. Amer. Vet. Med. Ass.* **142,** 502.

McLean, A. E. M., and Magee, P. N. (1970). *Brit. J. Exp. Pathol.* **51,** 587.

Magee, P. N. (1956). *Biochem. J.* **64,** 676.

Magee, P. N. (1958). *Biochem. J.* **70,** 606.

Magee, P. N. (1969). *Ann. N.Y. Acad. Sci.* **163,** 717.

Magee, P. N. (1971). *Food Cosmet, Toxicol.* **9,** 207.

Magee, P. N., and Barnes, J. M. (1956). *Brit. J. Cancer* **10,** 114.

Magee, P. N., and Barnes, J. M. (1959). *Acta Unio Int. Contra Cancrum* **15,** 187.

Magee, P. N., and Barnes, J. M. (1962). *J. Pathol. Bacteriol.* **84,** 19.

Magee, P. N., and Barnes, J. M. (1967). *Advan. Cancer Res.* **10,** 163.

Magee, P. N., and Farber, E. (1962). *Biochem. J.* **83,** 114.

Magee, P. N., and Hultin, T. (1962). *Biochem. J.* **83,** 106.

Magee, P. N., and Schoental, R. (1964). *Brit. Med. J.* **20,** 102.

Magee, P. N., and Swann, P. F. (1969). *Brit. Med. Bull.* **25,** 240.

Magee, P. N., and Vandekar, M. (1958). *Biochem. J.* **70,** 600.

Malins, D. C., Roubal, W. T., and Robisch, P. A. (1970). *J. Agr. Food Chem.* **18,** 740.

Manning, P. B., Coulter, S. T., and Jenness, R. (1968). *J. Dairy Sci.* **51,** 1725.

Marquardt, H., Schwaier, R., and Zimmermann, F. (1963a). *Naturwissenschaften* **50,** 135.

Marquardt, H., Zimmermann, F. K., and Schwaier, R. (1963b). *Naturwissenschaften* **50,** 625.

Marquardt, H., Zimmermann, F. K., and Schwaier, R. (1964). *Z. Vererbungslehre* **95,** 82.

Marquardt, P., and Hedler, L. (1966). *Arzneim.-Forsch.* **16,** 778.

Meijer, W. (1963). "Food Additive Control in the Netherlands." United Nations (FAO), Rome.

Miller, J. A. (1964). *Fed. Proc., Fed. Amer. Soc. Exp. Biol.* **23,** 1361.

Mirvish, S. S. (1970). *J. Nat. Cancer Inst.* **44,** 633.

Mirvish, S. S. (1971a). *J. Nat. Cancer Inst.* **46,** 1183.

Mirvish, S. S. (1971b). *

Mizrahi, I. J., and Emmelot, P. (1962). *Cancer Res.* **22,** 339.

Mizrahi, I. J., and Emmelot, P. (1963). *Biochem. Pharmacol.* **12,** 55.

Moehler, K., and Mayrhofer, O. L. (1968). *Z. Lebensm-Unter.-Forsch.* **135,** 313.

Moehler, K., and Mayrhofer, O. L. (1969). *Eur. Meet. Meat Res. Workers, 15th, 1969* p. 302.

Mohr, U., and Althoff, J. (1965). *Z. Naturforsch. B* **20,** 501.

Mohr, U., Althoff, J., and Wrba, H. (1965). *Gynaecologia* **160,** 381.

Mohr, U., Althoff, J., and Authaler, A. (1966). *Cancer Res.* **26,** 2349.

Montesano, R., and Magee, P. N. (1970). *Nature (London)* **228,** 173.

Montesano, R., and Saffiotti, U. (1968). *Cancer Res.* **28,** 2197.

Napalkov, N. P., and Alexandrov, V. A. (1968). *Z. Krebsforsch.* **71,** 32.

Navarro, F., Rodriguez, A., and Sancho, J. (1962). *An. Real Soc. Espan. Fis. Quim., Ser. B* **58,** 571.

Neurath, G., Pirman, B., and Wichern, H. (1964). *Beitr. Tabakforsch.* **2,** 311.

Neurath, G., Pirman, B., Leuttich, W., and Wichern, H. (1965). *Beitr. Tabakforsch,* **3,** 251.

Neurath, H. (1971). *

Noller, C. R. (1957). *In* "Chemistry of Organic Compounds," 2nd ed., p. 239. Saunders, Philadelphia, Pennsylvania.

Norris, E. R., and Benoit, G. J. (1945). *J. Biol. Chem.* **158,** 435.

Ogasawara, T., Ito, K., and Abe, N. (1963). *Nippon Nogei Kagaku Kaishi* **37,** 208; *Chem. Abstr.* **62,** 12375–12376 (1965).

O'Leary, J. F., Willis, J. H., Harrison, B., and Oikemus, A. (1957). *Proc. Soc. Exp. Biol. Med.* **94,** 775.

Orgeron, J. D., Martin, J. D., Caraway, C. T., Martine, R. M., and Hauser, G. H. (1957). *U.S. Pub. Health Rep.* **72,** 189.

Osswald, H., and Schmaehl, D. (1966). *Naturwissenschaften* **53,** 255.

Pasternak, L. (1964). *Arzneim.-Forsch.* **14,** 802.

Petrowitz, H. J. (1968). *Arzneim.-Forsch.* **18,** 1486.

Phillips, W. E. J. (1968a). *Can. Inst. Food Technol., J.* **1,** 98.

Phillips, W. E. J. (1968b). *J. Agr. Food Chem.* **16,** 88.

Pivnick, H., Rubin, L. J., Barnett, H. W., Nordin, H. R., Ferguson, P. A., and Perrin, C. H. (1967). *Food Technol.* **21,** 204.

Preussmann, R., Daiber, D., and Hengy, H. (1964a). *Nature (London)* **201,** 502.

Preussmann, R., Neurath, G., Wulf-Lorentzen, G., Daiber, D., and Hengy, H. (1964b). *Z. Anal. Chem.* **202,** 187.

Rao, C. N. R. (1963). "Chemical Applications of Infrared Spectroscopy," p. 275. Academic Press, New York.

Reay, G. A. (1938). *Annu. Rep. Food Invest. Bd. (Gt. Brit.)* p. 69.

Reay, G. A., and Shewan, J. M. (1951). *Advan. Food Res.* **2,** 343.

Reay, G. A., Cutting, C. L., and Shewan, J. M. (1943). *J. Soc. Chem. Ind., London* **62,** 77.

Reuber, M. D., and Lee, C. W. (1968). *J. Nat. Cancer Inst.* **41,** 1133.

Rhoades, J. W., and Johnson, D. E. (1970). *J. Chromatogr. Sci.* **8,** 616.

Richardson, W. D. (1907). *J. Amer. Chem. Soc.* **29,** 1757.

Roberts, J. D., and Caserio, M. C. (1964). "Basic Principles of Organic Chemistry," pp. 656–666. Benjamin, New York.

Saito, K., and Sameshima, M. (1956). *J. Agr. Chem. Soc. Jap.* **30,** 353.

Sakshaug, J., Soegnen, E., Aas Hansen, M., and Koppang, N. (1965). *Nature (London)* **206,** 1261.

Sander, J. (1967a). *Arch. Hyg. Bakteriol.* **151,** 22.

Sander, J. (1967b). *Hoppe-Seyler's Z. Physiol. Chem.* **348,** 852.

Sander, J. (1968). *Hoppe-Seyler's Z. Physiol. Chem.* **349,** 429.

Sander, J., and Schweinsberg, F. (1971). *

Sander, J., and Seif, F. (1969). *Arzneim.-Forsch.* **19,** 1091.

Sander, J., Schweinsberg, F., and Menz, H.-P. (1968). *Hoppe-Seyler's Z. Physiol Chem.* **349,** 1691.

Sander, J., Buerkle, G., Flohe, L., and Aeikens, B. (1971). *Arzneim.-Forsch.* **21,** 411.

Sasaki, A. (1938). *Tohoku J. Exp. Med.* **34,** 561.

Scanlan, R. A., and Libbey, L. M. (1971). *J. Agr. Food Chem.* **19,** 570.

Schmaehl, D., and Osswald, H. (1967). *Experientia* **23,** 497.

Schmaehl, D., and Preussmann, R. (1959). *Naturwissenschaften* **46,** 175.

Schmaehl, D., and Thomas, C. (1965). *Z. Krebsforsch.* **66,** 533.

Schoental, R. (1960). *Nature (London)* **188,** 420.

Schoental, R. (1961). *Nature (London)* **192,** 670.

Schoental, R. (1966). *Nature (London)* **209,** 148.

Schulz, M. E., Kay, H., and Mrowetz, G. (1960). *Milchwissenschaft* **15,** 556.

Schuphan, W. (1965). *Z. Ernaehrungswiss.* **5,** 207.

Schwarz, G., and Thomasow, J. (1950). *Milchwissenschaft* **5,** 376 and 412.

Sen, N. P. (1970). *J. Chromatogr.* **51,** 301.

Sen, N. P. (1971). *

Sen, N. P. (1972). *Food Cosmet. Toxicol.* **10,** 219.

Sen, N. P., and Dalpé, C. (1972). *Analyst* **97,** 216.

Sen, N. P., Smith, D. C., Schwinghamer, L., and Marleau, J. J. (1969a). *J. Ass. Offic. Anal. Chem.* **52,** 47.

Sen, N. P., Smith, D. C., and Schwinghamer, L. (1969b). *Food Cosmet. Toxicol.* **7,** 301.

Sen, N. P., Smith, D. C., Schwinghamer, L., and Howsam, B. (1970). *Can. Inst. Food Technol., J.* **3,** 66.

Serfontein, W. J., and Hurter, P. (1966). *Cancer Res.* **26,** 575.

Shewan, J. M. (1937a). *Annu. Rep. Food Invest. Bd. (Gt. Brit.)* p. 79.

Shewan, J. M. (1937b). *Annu. Rep. Food Invest. Bd. (Gt. Brit.)* p. 75.

Shewan, J. M. (1938). *In* "Report of the Director of Food Investigation for the Year 1938," pp. 79–87. HM Stationery Office, London.

Shewan, J. M. (1951). *Biochem. Soc. Symp.* **6,** 28.

Silliker, J. H., Greenberg, R. A., and Schack, W. R. (1958). *Food Technol.* **12,** 551.

Sinclair, K. B., and Jones, D. I. H. (1964). *J. Sci. Food Agr.* **15,** 717.

Sinios, A., and Wodsak, W. (1965). *Deut. Med. Wochenschr.* **90,** 1856.

Spencer, R. (1970). *In* "The Occurrence of Nitrate and Nitrites in Foods" (compiled by R. Aston), pp. 1–13. Brit. Food Mfg. Ind. Res. Ass., Leatherhead, Surrey, England.

Stenberg, A. I., Shillinger, Y. I., and Shevchenko, M. G. (1969). "Food Additive Control in the U.S.S.R." United Nations (FAO), Rome.

Steyn, D. G. (1960). The problem of methaemoglobinemia due to nitrate-contaminated water. *Amer. J. Pub. Health* **41,** 986.

Stieglitz, E. J., and Palmer, A. E. (1934). *J. Pharmacol. Exp. Ther.* **51,** 398.

Sundsvold, O. C., Uppstad, B., Ferguson, G. W., McLachlan, T., and Feeley, D. (1969). *Tidsskr. Hermetikind.* **55,** 94.

Swann, P. F., and McLean, A. E. M. (1968). *Biochem. J.* **107,** 14P.

Tarr, H. L. A. (1939). *J. Fish. Res. Bd. Can.* **4,** 367.

Tarr, H. L. A. (1940). *J. Fish. Res. Bd. Can.* **5,** 187.

Tarr, H. L. A. (1969). *Can. Inst. Food Technol., J.* **2,** 42.

Tarr, H. L. A., and Sunderland, P. A. (1939). *Fish. Res. Bd. Can., Progr. Rep. Pac. Coast Sta.* No. 39, p. 13.

Tarr, H. L. A., and Sunderland, P. A. (1940a). *J. Fish. Res. Bd. Can.* **5,** 148.

Tarr, H. L. A., and Sunderland, P. A. (1940b). *Fish. Res. Bd. Can., Progr. Rep. Pac. Coast. Sta.* No. 44, p. 16.

Tarr, H. L. A., and Sunderland, P. A. (1940c). *J. Fish. Res. Bd. Can.* **5,** 36.

Taylor, T. W. J., and Price, L. S. (1929). *J. Chem. Soc., London* p. 2052.

Telling, G. M., Bryce, T. A., and Althorpe, J. (1971). *J. Agr. Food Chem.* **19,** 937.

194 N. P. Sen

Terracini, B., Palestro, G., Ramella, M., Gigliardi, R., and Montesano, R. (1966). *Brit. J. Cancer* **20**, 871.
Terracini, B., Magee, P. N., and Barnes, J. M. (1967). *Brit. J. Cancer* **21**, 559.
Thewlis, B. H. (1967). *Food Cosmet. Toxicol.* **5**, 333.
Thewlis, B. H. (1968). *Food Cosmet. Toxicol.* **6**, 822.
Thomas, C., and Bollmann, R. (1968). *Z. Krebsforsch.* **71**, 129.
Thomasow, J. (1947). *Milchwissenschaft* **2**, 354.
Tokunga, T. (1964). *Bull. Hokkaido Reg. Fish. Res. Lab.* **39**, 108.
Tolstikov, G. A., Jemilev, U. M., Jurjev, V. P., Gershanov, F. B., and Rafikov, S. R. (1971). *Tetrahedron Lett.* No. 30, p. 2807.
Tomiyasu, Y., and Zenitani, B. (1957). *Advan. Food Res.* **7**, 41.
Toth, B., Magee, P. N., and Shubik, P. (1964). *Cancer Res.* **24**, 1712.
Tozawa, H., Enokihara, K., and Amano, K. (1969). "Proposed Modification of Dyer's Method for Trimethylamine Determination in Cod Fish," Tech. Conf. Fish Inspection and Quality Control, p. 1, FAO, Halifax, N.S.
Trams, A., and Kuenkel, H. A. (1964). *Biophysik* **1**, 422.
Uhl, E., and Hansen, S. C. (1961). "Food Additive Control in Denmark." United Nations, (FAO) Rome.
U.K. Food Additive Regulations (1962). The Preservatives in Food Regulations, H.M. Stationery Office, London.
U.S. Food Additive Regulations (1972). Code of Federal Regulations. Office of the Federal Register, Washington, D.C.
Van Ginkel, J. G. (1969). Presented at the 12th Session of the Committee of Government Experts on the Code of Principles Concerning Milk and Milk Products. Joint FAO/WHO Food Standards Program, Rome.
Veleminsky, J., and Gichner, T. (1968). *Mutat. Res.* **5**, 429.
Venkatesan, N., Arcos, J. C., and Argus, M. F. (1968). *Life Sci.* **7**, 1111.
Venkatesan, N., Argus, M. F., and Arcos, J. C. (1970a). *Cancer Res.* **30**, 2556.
Venkatesan, N., Arcos, J. C., and Argus, M. F. (1970b). *Cancer Res.* **30**, 2563.
Vesselinovitch, S. D. (1969). *Cancer Res.* **29**, 1024.
Wada, M. (1930). *Biochem. Z.* **224**, 420.
Walters, C. L. (1971). *Lab. Pract.* **20**, 574.
Walters, C. L., Johnson, E. M., and Ray, N. (1970). *Analyst* **95**, 485.
Walters, C. L., Saxby, M. J., and Newton, B. E. (1971). *
Walton, G. (1951). *Amer. J. Pub. Health* **41**, 986.
Watson, D. W. (1939). *J. Fish. Res. Bd. Can.* **4**, 267.
Watts, B. M. (1954). *Advan. Food Res.* **5**, 20.
Weckel, K. G., and Chien, S. (1969). "Use of Sodium Nitrite in Smoked Great Lakes Chub," Res. Rep. No. 51. College of Agricultural and Life Sciences, University of Wisconsin, Madison.
Weisburger, J. H., Weisburger, E. K., Mantel, N., Hadiadin, Z., and Fredrickson, T. (1966). *Naturwissenschaften* **53**, 508.
Weurman, C., and DeRooy, C. (1961). *J. Food Sci.* **26**, 239.
Wick, E. L., Underriner, E., and Paneras, E. (1967). *J. Food Sci.* **32**, 365.
Wilson, J. K. (1943). *J. Amer. Soc. Agron.* **35**, 279.
Woerner, F., and Fricker, A. (1960). *Deut. Molkerei Ztg.* **81**, 1345.

AUTHOR INDEX

Numbers in italics refer to the pages on which the complete references are listed.

SUBJECT INDEX

A

Abramis, roe toxin of, 101
Abramis brama, see Abramis
Acenaphthalene, in mutton, 9
Acetylglucosaminidase, in egg white, 43
Acipenser sturio, see Sturgeon
Additives, food 2–5
Adrenaline, in cheese, 23
Aflatoxin
  in meat, 10
  in milk, 23
Ageneiosus armatus, see Catfish
Albumin, egg, 25, 26
Alewife, trimethylamme oxide in, 143
Algae, 112–116, 123–128, *see also* individual species
  blue-green, 125–128
  geographic distribution of, 114, 115
  toxins produced by, 112–116, 126–128
  yellow-brown, 128
Alkylnitrosamines, metabolism of, 179
Alkylureas, nitrosation of, 151
Allergies, food, 31, 32
Amanita muscaria, see Mushrooms
Amines
  in cheese, 23, 145, 146
  in fish, 143
  interaction with nitrites, 146–151
  in milk, 146

Amino acids, nitrosation of, 147, 149
Amphibians, eggs of, 106
Anabaena flos-aquae, see also Algae
  toxins of, 125, 127
Anchovies, 105
Anemia, microcytic, 14
Anthracene
  in mutton, 9
  in steaks, charcoal-broiled, 10
Antibiotics
  in meat, 10
  in milk, 18
  as preservative, 3
Aphanizomenon flos-aquae, see also Algae, 127
Arabidopsis thaliana, effect of nitrosamines on, 178
Arothron
  hispidus, 78, 79, 87
  species of, 80, 81
Asthma, bronchial, due to milk intolerance, 14
Atherosclerosis, 26–29, 32
  role of cholesterol, 26, 27
  role of fats, 27, 28
  role of sugar, 28
  role of water hardness, 29
Avidin, 40, 42, 44, 48–55
  amino acid composition of, 44
  assay, 50–52
  denaturation of, 54

210